The Medical

Cannabis Guidebook

The Definitive Guide to Using and
Growing Medicinal Marijuana

by Jeff Ditchfield and Mel Thomas

Green Candy Press

Printed in China by Oceanic Graphic International

Sometimes Massively Distributed by P.G.W.

If a law is unjust, a man is not only right to disobey it; he is obligated to do so.

—Thomas Jefferson (1743-1826)

Contents

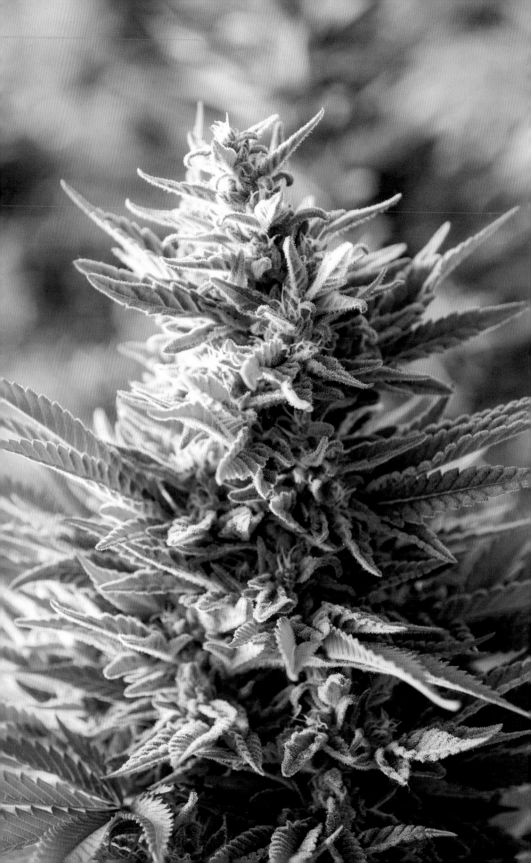

Why is Cannabis Illegal?

Referred to variously as marijuana, ganja, weed and herb amongst many other slang terms, cannabis is one of the safest medicines available. As well as giving us the dried buds that can be smoked, the plant produces nutritious seeds from which healthy edible oils can be pressed, the plant fibers are durable and versatile with many commercial uses, the crop is environmentally beneficial and many parts of the plant were in use for thousands of years before prohibition. Unlike many pharmaceutical medications, there has never been a single recorded fatality from cannabis use. No one has ever died as a direct result of ingesting cannabis, nor have there been any instances of brain receptor damage through its use; unlike alcohol and other drugs cannabis does not wear out the brain receptors, it merely stimulates them. One estimate of THC's lethal dose for humans indicates that 1500 pounds (680 kilograms) of cannabis would have to be smoked within 15 minutes (approximately) for the smoker to die. If you wanted to kill someone using 1500 pounds of cannabis you would be better advised to drop it on them.

LD50, also called median lethal dose, is the standard measure of the toxicity of a material through ingestion, skin contact or injection. LD50 is measured in micrograms (or milligrams) of the material per kilogram of the test-animal's body weight. The lower the amount, the more toxic the material. The estimated LD50 (lethal threshold) for cannabis, established in 1988 by the DEA's appropriate

---

Genus C.sativa has two main species, C. indica and C.ruderalis.

fact-finder, is 1:20,000 or 1:40,000. In layman's terms this means that in order to induce death a cannabis smoker would have to consume 20,000 to 40,000 times as much cannabis as is contained in one 0.9 gram joint.[1]

Studies indicate that the effective dose of THC is at least 1000 times lower than the estimated lethal dose (therapeutic ratio of 1000:1). Heroin has a therapeutic ratio of 6:1, alcohol and Valium both have a ratio of 10:1. Cocaine has a ratio of 15:1. Aspirin has a therapeutic ratio of 20:1; 20 times the recommended dose (40 tablets) can cause death and almost certainly induce extensive internal bleeding. Drugs used to treat patients with cancer, glaucoma and multiple sclerosis (MS) are all known to be highly toxic; the ratio of some drugs used in antineoplastic (cancer inhibiting) therapies have therapeutic ratios below 1.5:1.[2]

A small percentage of people may experience a negative or allergic reaction to cannabis use and a few patients suffer especially high heart rates and/or anxiety when being treated with cannabis oil, although this is a comparatively low number and the effects are merely unpleasant and cease when cannabis use is discontinued. Many bronchial asthma sufferers benefit from both herbal cannabis and cannabis oil extracts but for some it can serve as an additional irritant. However, for the overwhelming majority of people, cannabis has demonstrated literally hundreds of therapeutic uses.

So Why is There Almost Global Prohibition of this Plant?

Cannabis prohibition emanates from a commercial conspiracy that was started in the 1920s. The word *marijuana* itself was first brought into the English language by these early corporate offenders who needed to change the public's perception of the cannabis plant from a useful fiber and medicine to a dangerous, addictive and destructive substance in order to destroy the hemp industry and replace cannabis medicines and hemp fiber products with their own toxic pharmaceutical drugs and petrochemical products. They achieved this by manipulating the media and printing fictitious stories connecting marijuana use and crime. The manipulation continues to this day, as former CBS News president Richard Salant explained when discussing the media's role in manipulating the masses: "Our job is to give people not what they want, but what we decide they ought to have."[3]

Cannabis prohibition is indisputably the result of a corrupt conspiracy

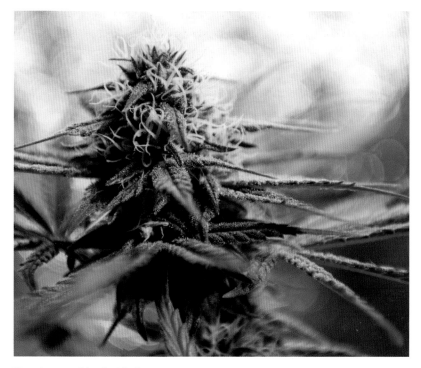

Female cannabis plant in flower.

founded on lies, propaganda and misinformation that for decades has denied society access to a benign and highly beneficial medicinal plant.

Cannabis has been used medically for millennia.[4] An article published in *The Economist* on April 27, 2006, under the heading, "Marijuana is medically useful, whether politicians like it or not," stated:

"If Marijuana was unknown, and bio-prospectors were suddenly to find it in some remote mountain crevice, its discovery would no doubt be hailed as a medical breakthrough. Scientists would praise its potential for treating everything from pain to cancer and marvel at its rich pharmacopoeia; many of whose chemicals mimic vital molecules in the human body."[5]

The medicinal use of cannabis predates written history. Cannabis preparations have traditionally been used as treatments for a wide variety of conditions for thousands of years in India, China, the Middle East, Southeast Asia, South Africa and South America. Furthermore, evidence of medicinal cannabis use dating from 1600 BCE has been found in Egypt, where it was used as a fumigant, topical salve and suppository.[6]

One of the earliest accounts of medical cannabis use can be found in the Chinese pharmacopoeia text *Pen-Tsao Kang-Mu* (*The Great Herbal*), which was written in 100 CE, but which actually dates back to the Emperor Shen-Nung in 2800 BCE.[7] The author Li Shih Chen referred to works from previous writers who for centuries regarded cannabis and its seeds as both a food and medicine. This early text correctly identifies the flowering tops of cannabis plants (*Ma-fen*) as the most useful and potent for the production of medicines, and recommends cannabis to treat menstrual fatigue, fevers, arthritis and malaria, as well as being effective as an analgesic. In the second century CE, Chinese surgeon Hua Tuo is documented as using an anesthetic made from cannabis resin and wine (*Ma-yo*) to perform painless complex surgical procedures, including limb amputations.

The Greek physician and botanist Pedanius Dioscorides traveled throughout the Roman and Greek empires to obtain material for his publication *Materia Medica,* which includes references to the plant *Cannabis Sativa L.* (from the Greek word *kannabis*), described as useful in the manufacturing of rope, with the juice of the seeds reported to be effective for treating earaches and diminishing sexual desire.[8] *Materia Medica* was translated and published throughout the known world and was used as a medical reference resource up until the 16th Century. It was a precursor to modern pharmacopoeias and is one of the most influential herbalist books ever written.

America's very first law concerning cannabis was enacted at Jamestown Colony, Virginia in 1619. Far from prohibiting cannabis, the law stated that all farmers were "ordered" to grow Indian hemp seed.[9] The U.S. Census of 1850 records 8,327 cannabis plantations in excess of 2,000 acres, all producing cannabis hemp for cloth, canvas and rope. Cannabis first appeared in the U.S. Pharmacopoeia in 1851 (3rd edition) and until prohibition was introduced, cannabis was the primary treatment for over 100 separate illnesses and diseases. By the time the 12th edition of the Pharmacopeia was published, cannabis had been officially removed and its use in medical research had been halted.

In the 1930s, the U.S. federal government backed the campaign of Harry Anslinger and his newly formed Bureau of Narcotics. Anslinger was a corrupt, racist bigot who in order to build up his new organization sought to generate fear of cannabis use through propaganda and lies. Anslinger created nationwide concern over a problem that did not exist by demonizing marijuana through spurious tales of crime, violence and insanity. The Bureau of Narcotics promoted

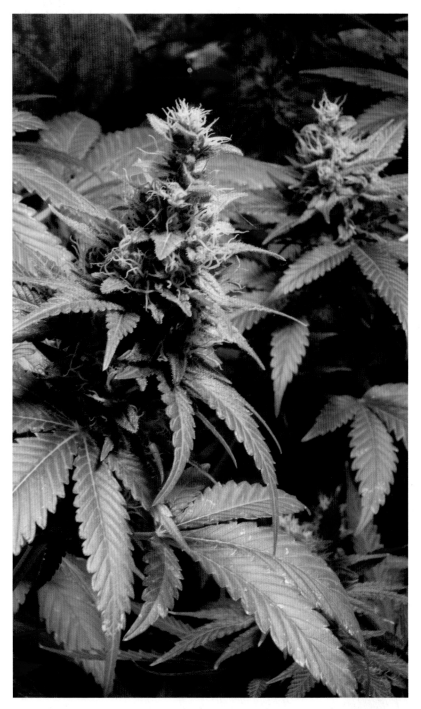

Plant in early stage of flowering.

what they called the "Gore Files"; wild "reefer madness" tales of murder, violence, loose morals and the effects cannabis had on the "degenerate races," which cynically exploited the endemic racism that was prevalent at the time. By associating marijuana use with ethnic minorities he ensured that the majority of white Americans would be sympathetic to any planned prohibition.

The Following Quotes Are From Anslinger's "Gore Files":

"There are 100,000 total marijuana smokers in the U.S., and most are Negroes, Hispanics, Filipinos, and entertainers. Their Satanic music, jazz, and swing, result from marijuana use. This marijuana causes white women to seek sexual relations with Negroes, entertainers, and any others."[10]

"...the primary reason to outlaw marijuana is its effect on the degenerate races."[11]

"Marijuana is an addictive drug which produces in its users insanity, criminality, and death."[12]

"Reefer makes darkies think they're as good as white men."[13]

"You smoke a joint and you're likely to kill your brother."[14]

"Marijuana is the most vio'ence-causing drug in the history of mankind."[15]

The Bureau of Narcotics had a powerful and willing ally in the media mogul William Randolph Hearst, who had invested heavily in the timber industry to support his chain of national newspapers. To Hearst, hemp paper was unwanted competition and he readily published lurid anti-cannabis propaganda from the Bureau's "Gore Files", printing headlines such as:

"Marihuana makes fiends of boys in thirty days - Hashish goads users to bloodlust."[16]

"Marihuana influenced negroes to look at white people in the eye, step on white men's shadows, and look at a white woman twice."

Drug Menace...

MARIJUANA

How an Innocent-Looking Plant, a Roadside Weed In Many States, Presents A Grave Narcotic Problem

By WILLIAM WOLF

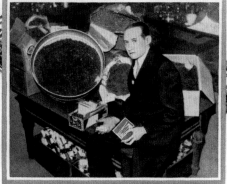

Some of the marijuana captured in a raid. The cigarettes often cost several dollars each

powerful narcotic effects when smoked. This probably occurred in Mexico.

Suddenly, the nation awoke to the fact that it had a major drug problem on its hands. Marijuana smoking, which was confined at first to Mexico and the Southwestern States, started to spread. And, worst of all, the plant from which the narcotic came not only could be grown anywhere, but actually was growing wild in many states!

Early this year, a house was raided in a small New Jersey town, and marijuana worth $6,000 was seized. The person arrested had in his possession a large quantity of the dried and prepared weed. He confessed that it was grown on a small plot of ground belonging to the house he rented.

The commercial production of marijuana is as simple as that—a field is planted and the weed grows. It needs no special preparation before being sold as a drug, other than drying the leaves and flowers. The only thing that led to this arrest was a quarrel with somebody who knew what the "patch of weeds" was and told police officials about the secret back-yard crop.

Federal authorities reported last fall at the end of the growing season that large acreages of *Cannabis sativa* were destroyed in Pennsylvania, New York, Ohio, California, and Georgia. At the same time, evidence of its widespread cultivation was contained in the additional report that, within a few days' time, investigations and seizures were made at points as widely separated as Rochester, N. Y., Fremont, Ohio, Sacramento, Calif., and Columbus, Ga.

Because it was circulated so generally in this nation's early history, marijuana now is a roadside weed in many sections of the country.

For that reason, Federal authorities regard it as a puzzling problem. Furthermore, over fifteen states failed to adopt the uniform narcotic-drugs act under which the Federal authorities could prosecute peddlers and growers of the weed. Some of these states only forbid the importation of marijuana; and, since it grows anywhere, such laws obviously are useless.

Where it is grown for sale as "dope," considerable ingenuity is expended in concealing the fields containing it. In the Ohio case reported by Federal officials, a large stand of Indian hemp was hidden by surrounding cornfields. That is a favorite trick of growers, to hide the marijuana with higher-growing crops.

The average citizen can help stamp out marijuana by reporting to the proper authorities any suspicious growth hidden by corn, alfalfa, or similar crops. The weed grows four to eight feet or more in height, has a sticky surface when touched, and gives off a strong narcotic odor. When grown for its fiber, it is cut before reaching full growth; but when intended for illegal uses, it is allowed to blossom, since it is the flowering tops, the leaves, and the small stems that are gathered and dried for smoking.

The plant has erect, branching, and angular stems, while the leaves are alternate and opposite on long, lax footstalks. The leaves have sawlike edges and may be odd or even in number, but usually about eight leaves are in one group.

What are the (Continued on page 119)

A patch of Indian hemp found growing in the side yard of a San Francisco home. The occupant of the house was arrested

MAY, 1936

13

Anti-cannabis propaganda from 1936.

"Marihuana is responsible for the raping of white women by crazed negroes."

"Three fourths of the crimes of violence in this country today are committed by dope slaves, that is a matter of cold record."[17]

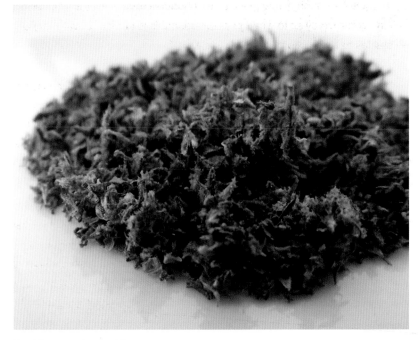

Freshly ground cannabis.

Hearst and Anslinger were joined in the conspiracy by the Dupont chemical corporation, and in 1937 Anslinger presented to Congress his Marijuana Tax Act.[18] Apart from some opposition from William C. Woodward of the American Medical Association, the bill was passed after very little discussion, and cannabis was effectively prohibited. Most people did not realize that the "evil marijuana drug" that was referred to in the tax act was in fact the cannabis plant that had been essential to the early settlers and was a useful and well-known medicine.

Due to the racist corruption surrounding the use of the name "marijuana," from here onward we will call this plant by its correct name: cannabis.

Today, there is renewed interest in the medical use of cannabis, with numerous respected doctors and scientists researching its many and varied indicators. A study sponsored by the State of California, conducted by the University of California Center for Medicinal Cannabis Research, and published in *The Open Neurology Journal* (September 2012), concluded that cannabis provides much-needed relief to chronic pain sufferers and that more clinical trials are desperately needed:

"The classification of marijuana as a Schedule I drug as well as the continuing controversy as to whether or not cannabis is of medical value are obstacles to medical progress in this area..."[19]

"Based on evidence currently available the Schedule I classification is not tenable; it is not accurate that cannabis has no medical value, or that information on safety is lacking. It is true cannabis has some abuse potential, but its profile more closely resembles drugs in Schedule III. The continuing conflict between scientific evidence and political ideology will hopefully be reconciled in a judicious manner."

Multinational pharmaceutical companies are now growing tons of cannabis plants at secret, heavily guarded locations, in order to extract just two of the plant's cannabinoids, mix them with alcohol, glycerin and a small amount of peppermint for flavor, and market the end product as a "mucosal" spray (which means you basically squirt it under your tongue) called Sativex.

Sativex Spray

This cannabis-based product was developed by GW Pharmaceuticals in the United Kingdom at heavily guarded farms where they grow over 20 tons of cannabis annually. This is then processed and the cannabinoids THC and CBD are extracted to be made into an alcohol-based tincture. They charge patients around $190.00 (approximately) per 10-milliliter vial, which is only enough to last the average multiple sclerosis (MS) patient 10 days. [20] There are estimated to be 80,000 MS sufferers in the U.K. alone; you do the math. If patients were allowed to grow their own cannabis they could produce a generic copy of Sativex for $8 per 10 milliliters. The authors have actually proved this and demonstrated the product at cannabis conventions in both Barcelona and Valencia in 2013. There is a video taken at *Spannabis* in Barcelona on their website (cannabiscure.info) that verifies this.

Regardless of the enormous profits being made at the expense of sick people, cannabis buds and oil are far superior to Sativex as you benefit from the full and complex profile of cannabinoids, not just THC and CBD. In addition, patients don't experience any ulcers, burning sensations in the mouth or the unpleasant aftertaste of alcohol that many who use Sativex complain of.

In U.S. states such as California and Colorado, cannabis can be purchased at state-sanctioned dispensaries, but according to the Controlled Substances Act, cannabis is a Schedule I drug, listed alongside dangerous narcotics. The American Chronic Pain Society says in *ACPA Medications & Chronic Pain, Supplement 2007:*

"Some states allow the legal use of marijuana for health purposes including pain, while the federal government continues to threaten physicians with prosecution for prescribing it."[21]

There have been two rulings since 2001, United States v. Oakland Cannabis Buyers Cooperative and Gonzales v. Raich, which have confirmed the federal government's commitment to prosecuting buyers and sellers even in states where cannabis has been approved for medical use.[22, 23] The FDA's official stance on cannabis states:

"Marijuana has a high potential for abuse, has no currently accepted medical use in treatment in the United States, and has a lack of accepted safety for use under medical supervision."[24]

Despite this fallacious statement, Sativex is licensed to Otsuka Pharmaceutical Co., Ltd. in the United States as a treatment for spasticity resulting from multiple sclerosis (MS), and as a possible treatment for the side effects from conventional cancer therapies.[25] Furthermore, synthetic cannabinoids such as Nabilone and Cesamet are available as prescription drugs in many countries.[26, 27] These synthetic copies of cannabinoids are expensive and compare poorly to cannabis plant extracts.

In April 2011, GW Pharmaceuticals entered into an exclusive license agreement for Novartis Pharma AG to commercialize Sativex in Australia, New Zealand, Asia and Africa.[28] Under the agreement, GW Pharmaceuticals received an upfront payment of $5 million and is eligible for additional payments totaling $28.75 million upon the achievement of set commercial sales targets. In addition, GW Pharmaceuticals will receive royalties on all net sales.[29] In 2009, the global pharmaceutical industry market was valued at $837 billion and estimated to reach $1 trillion by 2014.[30]

The profits for pharmaceutical companies targeting the cancer market expanded to $24 billion in 2004, with the highest growth rates occurring in the

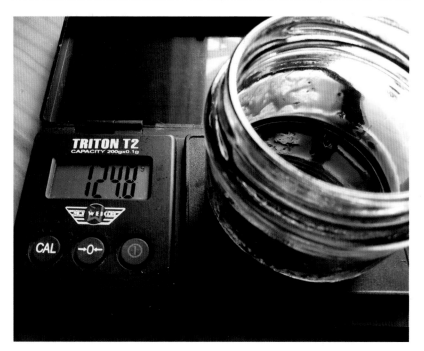

Cannabis oil.

antineoplastic (cancer inhibiting) class of drugs.[31] The market for these drugs was valued at around $43 billion in 2005 and $69 billion in 2010.[32] Why would these multinational corporations be interested in researching and promoting a cancer treatment that can be grown for free and is difficult to effectively patent unless kept illegal?

The following multiple-medicinal-use patent on a natural compound, which is illegal under patent statutes, was recently granted to the U.S. government by its own Patent Office:

Excerpt from U.S. Patent #6630507:[33]

"Cannabinoids have been found to have antioxidant properties, unrelated to NMDA receptor antagonism. This new found property makes cannabinoids useful in the treatment and prophylaxis of a wide variety of oxidation associated diseases, such as ischemic, age-related, inflammatory and autoimmune diseases. The cannabinoids are found to have particular application as neuro-protectants, for example in limiting neurological damage following ischemic insults, such as stroke and trauma, or in the treatment of neurodegenerative diseases, such as Alzheimer's disease, Parkinson's disease and HIV dementia. Non-psychoactive cannabinoids, such as cannabidiol, are particularly advantageous to use because they avoid toxicity that is encountered with psychoactive cannabinoids at high doses useful in the method of the present invention. A particular disclosed class of cannabinoids useful as neuro-protective antioxidants is formula (I) wherein the R group is independently selected from the group consisting of H, CH_3, and $COCH_3$."

This is a complete contradiction to the U.S. government's officially stated policy with regard to medical cannabis use and clearly demonstrates that cannabis prohibition is not about protecting health–it's about protecting corporate wealth.

Apart from the nutritional and health benefits gained from non-psychoactive hemp seed and oils now legally available, there is overwhelming evidence that cannabis oil made from the illegal plant varieties can send many cancers into remission, particularly with regard to breast cancer. The antitumor effects of herbal cannabis and cannabis oil extracts have been well known since at least the 1970s, when the Medical College of Virginia reported on August 18, 1974, that marijuana's psychoactive component, THC, slowed the growth of lung cancers, breast cancers and a virus-induced leukemia in laboratory mice, and prolonged their lives by as much as 36%.[34] Funded by the National Institutes of Health and tasked with finding evidence that cannabis damages the immune system, the study instead found that THC slowed the growth of these three types of cancer: The Drug Enforcement Agency (DEA) quickly shut down the Virginia study and all further research was halted.

In 1998, a research team at Madrid's Complutense University discovered that THC could selectively induce programmed death in brain tumor cells without negatively impacting surrounding healthy cells.[35] Further studies reported in the August 15, 2004 issue of Cancer Research, the journal of the American Association for Cancer Research, that cannabis constituents inhibited the spread of brain cancer in human tumor biopsies.[36]

Led by Dr. Manuel Guzman, the Spanish team announced they had destroyed incurable brain cancer tumors in rats by injecting them with THC. This work still continues and the authors recently supplied the team with a quantity of their laboratory tested 1:1 (THC:CBD) oil containing 40% CBD with total active cannabinoids at 80%. This oil was made using the techniques described in this book, in later chapters, and research has shown that CBD (cannabidiol)–a nontoxic, non-psychoactive chemical compound found in the cannabis plant–acts as a more potent inhibitor of cancer cell growth than other cannabinoids, including THC. The compound is particularly efficacious in halting the spread of breast cancer cells by triggering apoptosis (programmed cell death).

Scientists at California Pacific Medical Center in San Francisco have also shown that CBD, can stop metastasis in many kinds of aggressive cancers, stating:[37]

> "We started by researching breast cancer, but now we've found that cannabidiol works with many kinds of aggressive cancers; brain, prostate and any kind in which these high levels of ID-1 are present."

Even if only anecdotal evidence exists regarding the efficacy of cannabis oil treatment on cancerous tumors in patients, then surely every cancer sufferer has the right to be informed about this and given the opportunity to try it. This is not a personal freedom argument but a discussion regarding the fundamental human right to life. Access to a potentially life-saving medication should not be subject to any laws whatsoever. People denied cannabis oil treatment have died of cancers that all of the available evidence suggests may have been entirely treatable. In the following chapters we'll look at the basic history and makeup of the cannabis plant, how its beneficial contents can best be extracted and administered and we'll also detail the nutritional benefits that can be derived from non-psychoactive varieties available such as hemp seeds and cold pressed hemp oils. The aim is to help people make their own informed decisions regarding cannabis use, regardless of the government's refusal to supply this information or allow cannabis use.

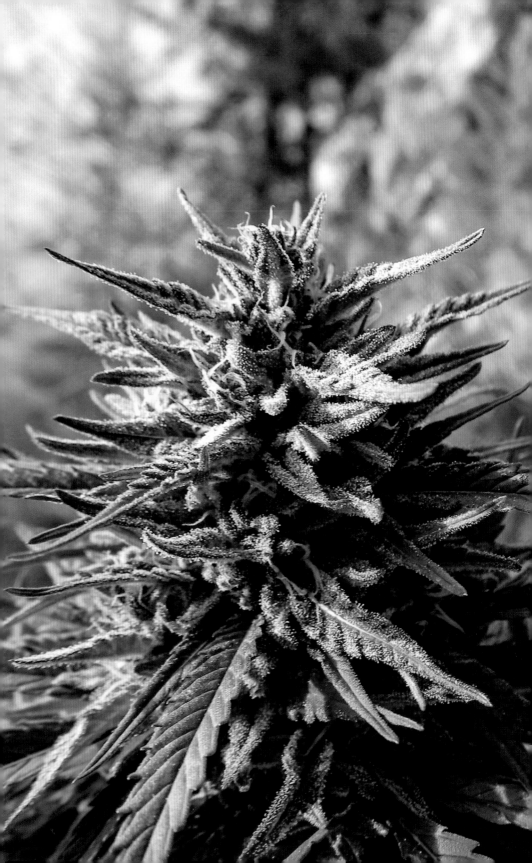

CHAPTER ONE

The Cannabis Plant

Cannabis sativa is a member of the Moraceae family and can grow to between 3 and 15 feet (1 and 4.5 meters), depending on the variety.[1] Landrace is the term used to describe a wild-growing cannabis strain that has evolved in the isolation of a specific geographic region. Over time, these isolated strains began to evolve their own distinct traits best suited for survival in their region. Cannabis strains as we know them today are the result of crossbreeding and hybridization of these distinct landraces.

Hemp is the common name for plants of the entire genus *C. sativa,* although the term now refers only to cannabis strains cultivated for fiber and not drug crops. Botanists still cannot agree as to which family cannabis belongs; initially, it was classified as one of the Nettle family (*Urticaceae*), although this was based more upon visual characteristic. It was later reclassified into the Fig family (*Moraceae*). However, this is still causing disagreement, so cannabis is now classified as *Cannabaceae*, along with the genus of hop plants. In most studies, hemp and hops are not separated from each other, but are reported as hops/hemp or *Cannabaceae*.[2]

Cannabis is dioecious; meaning that the plant will be either male or female. In unusual circumstances it can develop into a hermaphrodite (monoecious) plant; this means that both male and female flowers appear on the same plant. Only the female produces flowers containing significant amounts of

Maturing cannabis flower.

1

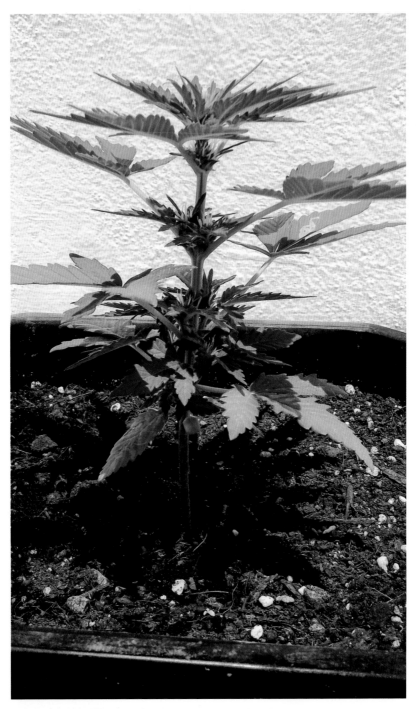

Young cannabis plant.

cannabinoids. These flowers are referred to as "buds" and they are more potent if the female is unfertilized by the male. These flowers are also known as sensimilla, meaning seedless in Spanish. Males and hermaphrodites are of no use to the medical or recreational cannabis consumer so growers must ensure that they cultivate only female plants by either taking cuttings from an established female mother plant or by starting the crop with feminized seeds to guarantee an all-female crop.

To regulate its development, the plant reads the amount of light it receives using a hormone called phytochrome, which acts as a photoreceptor, and is basically a pigment that plants use to detect light. When a cannabis plant receives over 12 hours of uninterrupted daylight, it deduces that it is early in the season and grows in what is referred to as the vegetative stage. This is when growth is focused on developing roots, branches and leaves. Once the amount of daylight falls below 12 hours, the plant changes its growth cycle into the flowering stage. This occurs naturally in the fall (autumn) as the plant prepares to breed and produce seeds for the following year, before dying back. Indoor growers can manipulate the light cycle without causing any problems to the plant by using timing switches on artificial lights that force the plant into thinking the season has changed. The flowering stage can be induced after as little as two weeks' vegetative growth. Outdoor growers can effect the same response in their plants by covering them or placing them in a dark room to ensure they are only receiving 12 hours of sunlight or less. There is no difference in the cannabinoid content of plants flowered after only two weeks' vegetative growth when compared to those given a longer vegetative period. The plants receiving the shorter period will simply be smaller and yield less.

There are three distinct cannabis drug varieties grown specifically for their compounds, a complex fusion of approximately 60 different cannabinoids and over 400 active components, principally THC (delta-9-tetrahydrocannabinol).[3] These are:

Cannabis Sativa

This landrace originates from equatorial regions and its plants can reach heights in excess of 15 feet (4.5 meters). They produce thin, spiky leaves and massive colas (where the flowers or buds grow together tightly) that are not very dense. Pure cannabis sativa strains are not generally used for indoor cul-

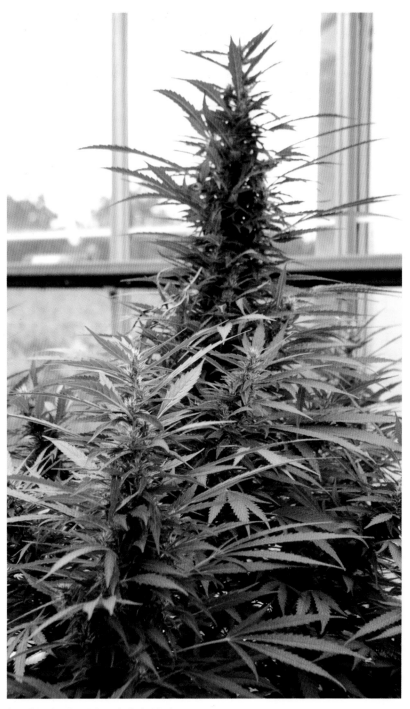

A sativa-dominant female hybrid plant.

tivation due to their size and maturation time. Cannabis sativa can take up four to eight times the space of a compact cannabis indica variety. There are now many hybrid varieties available for grow room cultivation, where the harvested flowers benefit from a high calyx-to-leaf ratio (meaning there are less leaves to trim from the finished buds).

Cannabis Indica

This landrace originates from the mountainous regions of Central Asia. Local strains were collected from Kashmir, Pakistan, Northern India and Nepal during the early 1960s and these native plants became the gene pool for many of today's varieties. They are characteristically stocky and hardy plants that produce broad, maple-like leaves and rarely reach heights in excess of 7 feet (2 meters) outdoors, producing heavy, tight flowers that are high in psychoactive content. Cannabis indica or indica-dominant hybrid plants are ideal for grow rooms and smaller medical cultivation set ups.

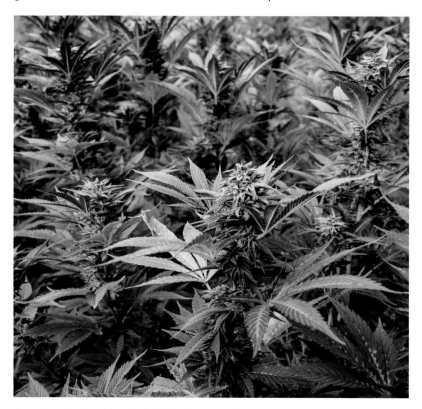

An indica-dominant female hybrid plant.

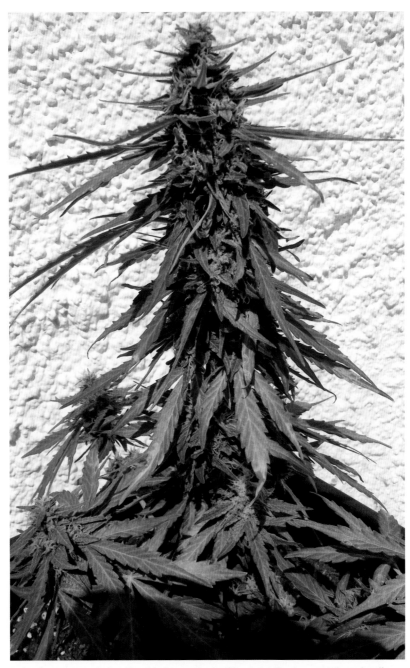

Auto-flowering varieties like this Lowryder by The Joint Doctor contain ruderalis genetics which means they do not require a "dark period" to induce flowering. They are the easiest varieties to cultivate. This particular plant was grown by Jeff in Spain.

Cannabis Ruderalis

This is a debated third landrace of cannabis found in Russia, Poland and other Eastern European countries. Schultes classified cannabis as having three species–sativa, indica, and ruderalis– based on the formation of the seed-pods. There is still some debate as to whether there is justification for this third category. The features of Cannabis ruderalis plants are large seeds and weedy plants around 5 feet (1.5 meters) tall that produce lower levels of THC than C. sativa or C. indica. However, it is a hardy plant that flowers early, in most cases regardless of the photoperiod. This auto-flowering gene has been bred into the strains of auto-flowers. Ruderalis flowers tend to be sparse and do not produce the same yields as other varieties, but it is a reasonable plant to use for medicinal cultivation as some strains can be high in CBD.

Auto-flowering plants are crossbreeds between cannabis ruderalis (which gives them the automatic flowering trait) and cannabis indica and/or cannabis sativa strains. These plants are not dependent on the light cycle to induce flowering; instead, the process triggers automatically when the particular strain is ready. This is generally a few weeks after planting, with a further five to seven weeks until harvest. The origins of auto-flowering cannabis plants are the subject of much debate, but one theory is that ruderalis genetics were introduced from a hybrid-cross of Mexican sativa and Russian ruderalis plants. Another theory is that the early genetics came from a Finnish hemp strain called Finola. Due to the lack of vegetative period, auto-flowerers produce smaller plants with a slightly lower THC content as a result of the cannabis ruderalis genetics, but they are hardy plants that are well suited to both indoor and outdoor cultivation.

Cannabis as a Crop

Reproduction in cannabis plants takes place when the male (staminate) pollen is united with the female (pistilate) cells. The stamen is simply the biological name given to the male plant's reproductive parts and the pistil is the name given to the female counterparts. Medicinal cannabis is principally grown for its flowering tops (also referred to as buds) and it is only the female plant that produces these. The male flower's sole purpose is to fertilize the female plants. Once the flowers open they disperse pollen, after which the plant dies back. As seeded buds are less desirable to medical and recreational consumers, knowledgeable cultivators identify any males in the crop and remove them, or

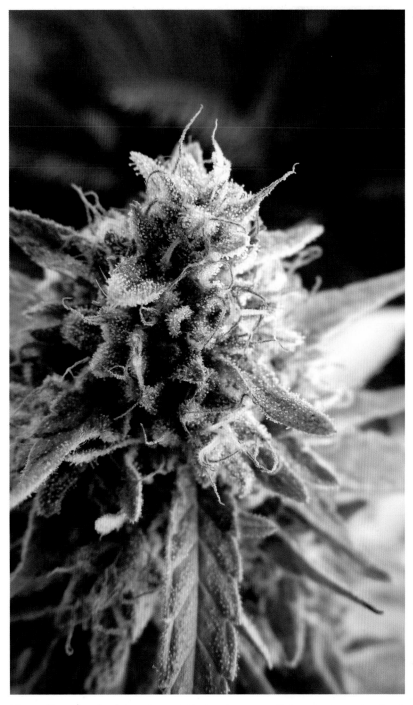

Mature flower nearing harvest.

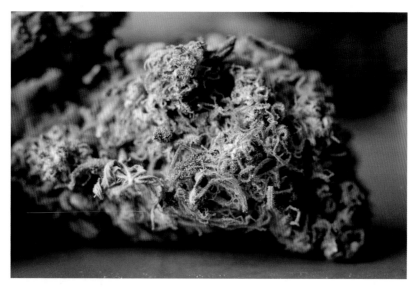

Dried, trimmed and cured bud.

cultivate crops of known females taken as cuttings from mother plants.

Of the 400 or more chemical compounds found in cannabis plants, the four main ones are delta-9-tetrahydrocannabinol (delta-9-THC), cannabidiol (CBD), delta-8-tetrahydrocannabinol and cannabinol (CBN).[4] Apart from cannabidiol, these compounds are all psychoactive, the most potent being delta-9-THC. Researchers from the University of Saskatchewan have discovered the chemical pathway that Cannabis sativa uses to create cannabinoids. Adjunct professor of biology Jon Page described the pathway as an unusual one that has never before been seen in plants, involving a specialized version of one enzyme called hexanoyl-CoA synthetase, and another enzyme called olivetolic acid cyclase (OAC).[5] The professor states: "What cannabis has done is take a rare fatty acid with a simple, six-carbon chain and use it as a building block to make something chemically complex and pharmacologically active."

Breeding and genetics define whether a cannabis strain is fiber hemp or has high cannabinoid content. Hemp grown for its fiber and seeds contains little THC, typically between 0.01% and 0.05% content compared to well over 15% in herbal cannabis grown for recreational or therapeutic use. Fiber hemp strains contain only trace amounts of psychoactive compounds and none of these are contained within the seeds, so in most parts of the world, hemp seeds and their oil are legally available from most good grocery stores and

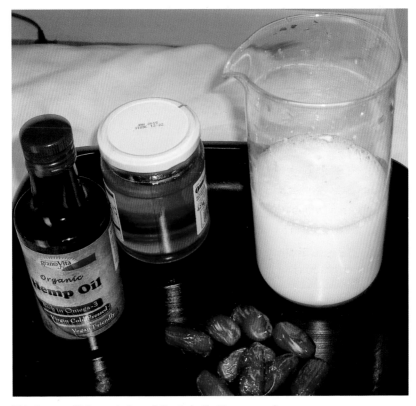

This hemp milk is made from fully de-hulled hemp seeds.

health food outlets. Hemp seed is one of nature's super foods; high in protein and vitamins, it also provides a broad spectrum of health benefits including improved digestion, increased and sustained energy levels, rapid recovery from sickness or injury, lowered cholesterol levels and reduced blood pressure, with an associated improvement in blood circulation and natural blood sugar control. Regular hemp seed has also been shown to boost the immune system and help to prevent illness.

Cannabis hemp seed oil contains gamma-linolenic acid (GLA), an omega-6 fatty acid that is found mainly in plant-based oils.[6] Omega-6 fatty acid is also known as polyunsaturated fatty acid (PUFA), one of the essential fatty acids.[7] These acids are necessary for optimum health, but the body doesn't naturally produce them. Along with omega-3 fatty acids, omega-6 fatty acids play a crucial role in brain function, as well as growth and development.[8] They help stimulate skin and hair growth, maintain bone strength and regulate the metabolism, and they play an important role in maintaining the reproductive system.

Fiber hemp is grown outdoors in dense rows to encourage tall, upward growth that produces very little foliage. Mature plants form a dense canopy that blocks light and helps choke weed growth, leaving the growing field in good condition the following season and substantially reducing the farm workload. Hemp is one of the fastest-growing biomass crops available; air-dried stem yields in Canada have ranged from 2.6 -14.0 tons of dry, retted stalks per hectare at 12% moisture (according to records dating back to 1998). Hemp produces some of the strongest and most versatile fibers known to man, which can be used to make products ranging from cloth to plastics. Its seeds are both a nutritious food and an excellent source of oil. The fiber from the stalk is still used in the modern production of fabrics such as canvas and linen, and also in the manufacture of specialty hemp papers, such as banknotes and high-quality printing paper.

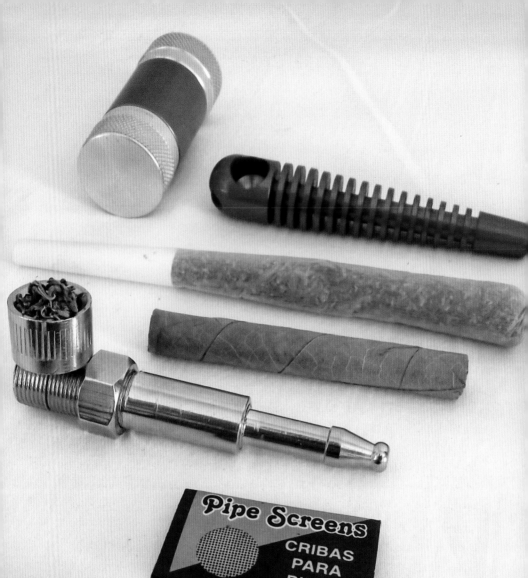

CHAPTER TWO

How Cannabis Works

Recreational and medicinal-quality psychoactive cannabis comes in several forms; herbal bud (dried flowering tops), resin (hash), kief, keef or kif (sometimes keif), which are the powdery resin glands (or trichomes), and oil. Referred to by many slang terms, cannabis is usually rolled into cigarettes known as a joints, but can also be smoked in a pipe, vaporized, made into milky or alcohol-based drinks and hot beverages, or eaten. If cannabis is smoked, the effects are normally felt within minutes; if eaten, the full effects can take up to an hour and are cumulative, often longer lasting and the uptake can be more variable.

When inhaled, cannabis compounds (cannabinoids) rapidly enter the bloodstream via the lungs, to be transported directly to the brain and other parts of the body. The feeling of being stoned or high is caused by the delta-9-THC binding to cannabinoid receptors in the brain.[1] There are also cannabinoid-like substances produced naturally by the brain itself, called endocannabinoids. Researchers at Hebrew University in Jerusalem identified the body's own form of THC, and christened the internally manufactured substance "anandamide" after the Sanskrit ananda, or bliss.[2] Most of these receptors are found in parts of the brain that influence pleasure, memory, thought, concentration and time perception. They are also involved in cognition, pain perception and motor coordination.

....

There are many ways to ingest cannabis.

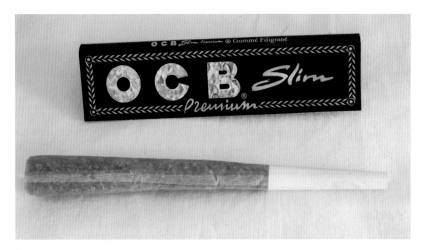

A pure cannabis joint containing no tobacco.

Around one in 10 people have reported unpleasant experiences at some point in their cannabis use, including confusion and anxiety. Interestingly, the same person may have either pleasant or unpleasant effects depending on their mood and circumstances. Side effects of cannabis use can include increased pulse rate, visual and sleep disturbance, decreased blood pressure, bloodshot eyes, dry mouth, increased appetite and mild lethargy. Heavy usage may possibly result in feelings of paranoia whilst under the influence. However, these side effects are temporary and pass quickly, mainly affecting people who have not used cannabis regularly. Cannabis consumers are therefore advised to accustom themselves to its use with smaller doses initially.

The most common effects of cannabis use are a sense of relaxation, happiness, sleepiness and an enhanced appreciation of external stimuli, with some consumers reporting that colors appear more intense. Many report becoming more animated, with a corresponding release of inhibitions, making them more talkative and humorous. Cannabis can also heighten sexual thoughts, desires and experiences. In India, cannabis has been used for thousands of years as an integral part of Tantric sex, which is not about sexual gratification, but rather devotion and worship; at the point of orgasm the devotee is said to be at one with the universe. Thought processes become enhanced and many philosophers, musicians, writers, poets and artists report using cannabis to increase their creativity. Many consumers report that listening to music and viewing artistic works become much more profound experiences whilst under the influence of cannabis.

The amount of time cannabis takes to be felt is dependent on the route of administration. Inhaling cannabis is the quickest way to administer a dose; vaporized or smoked cannabinoid material arrives in the lungs very quickly, entering the bloodstream and rapidly passing into the brain, and becomes active within minutes, with its effects lasting for several hours. If eaten, the cannabinoid compounds have to be absorbed from the stomach and then pass through the liver, where a percentage is metabolized into 11-Hydroxy-THC, which is four to five times more psychoactive than Delta9-THC.[3] It can take from 30 minutes to an hour to reach the brain, with the full effects taking up to three hours.

Cannabis as Medicine

Pharmaceutical cannabis sprays are designed for "mucosal or sublingual administration," meaning that the patient sprays it under their tongue, and the cannabinoids are then absorbed into the bloodstream via the mucus membrane.

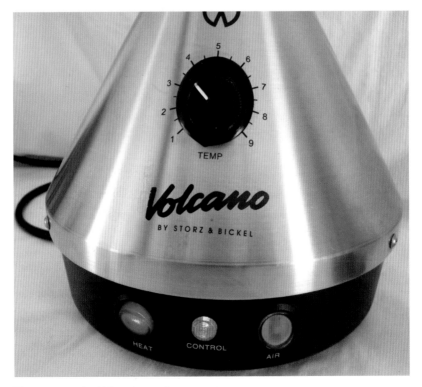

The very popular Volcano vaporizer.

This is quite an effective and convenient method of administration, which allows the cannabinoids to reach the brain within 10 to 20 minutes. However, a significant amount actually ends up being swallowed and absorbed through the gut, resulting in a sizable portion of the medication having a delayed onset. This is far from ideal for medical users who wish to accurately regulate their dosage. Many patients report that the pharmaceutical industry's expensive cannabis-based medications are vastly inferior to the natural product. Vaporizing organically grown cannabis buds is one of the most effective ways of self-medicating, particularly for pain relief.

For some patients the high associated with herbal cannabis use is undesirable. This is particularly true for those who need to medicate regularly throughout the day. One of the most useful cannabinoids is cannabidiol, or CBD, which unlike THC, binds poorly to the brain's receptors and can therefore work without getting patients stoned. A company in Safed, Israel called Tikun Olam began its research on CBD-enhanced cannabis strains in 2009. Recreational cannabis is illegal in Israel, but medicinal use has been permitted since 1993. It is used to treat over 9,000 people suffering from illnesses such as cancer, Parkinson's, multiple sclerosis, Crohn's disease and post-traumatic stress disorder. Tikun Olam has now developed a strain called Avidekel, which contains 15.8% CBD but less than 1% THC.[4] It remains to be seen how medical cannabis users will benefit from this strain, as the pharmaceutical companies making vast sums of money from their monopoly of cannabis-based medications will try to ensure that the general prohibition of cannabis continues so that patients can't legally grow their own Avidekel-type strains for vaporizing.

Commercially available strains that are high in CBD are now becoming more readily available specifically bred for medical use. One recommended seed company is the CBD Crew. The breeder behind this project is the renowned Shantibaba, who cofounded Mr. Nice seeds with Howard Marks. The authors produce their 1:1 (THC:CBD) 80% cannabinoid content oil using the CBD Crew's Skunk Haze strain. The highest CBD strain the authors have verified is known as Juanita La Lagrimosa and is produced by Reggae Seeds in Spain. This strain has been laboratory tested and gives consistent results; it comes in at a massive 8.81% CBD content with 6.77% THC. More information on these strains is available on the authors' website, cannabiscure.info.

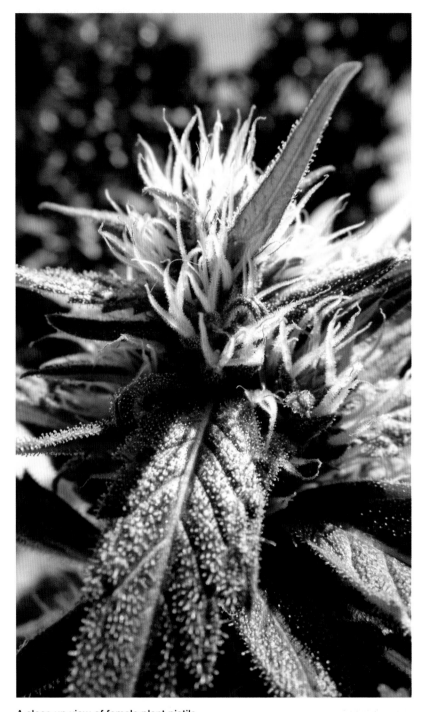

A close up view of female plant pistils.

Side Effects

A great deal of misinformation, unsupported by any reputable medical evidence, is quoted with regard to cannabis use and mental health issues. Starting in the 1920s, the prohibition conspiracy began with newspaper headlines and fabricated stories detailing what they termed "Reefer Madness." Today, the Partnership for a Drug Free America has a budget of around one million dollars a day, with the majority of their funding being provided by pharmaceutical companies who pay substantial sums of money to lobbyists and special interest groups to aggressively campaign against any possibility of cannabis legalization.[5] Cannabis does not cause mental health problems; there is no evidence to support this claim. If cannabis use caused mental illness, why would major pharmaceutical companies be marketing cannabinoid-based medications? Furthermore, if cannabis use caused schizophrenia there would be over 150,000,000 recreational users exhibiting an extraordinary range of symptoms worldwide. This is not the case. Professor David Nutt from the U.K. gave a lecture regarding cannabis and schizophrenia in 2009, referring to the idea that stronger cannabis (known as "Skunk", but not in reference to the strain of the same name) has made smoking cannabis more dangerous, and stated:

"Schizophrenia seems to be disappearing from the general population even though cannabis use has increased markedly in the last 30 years. When we were reviewing the general practice research database in the U.K. from the University of Keele, research consistently and clearly showed that psychosis and schizophrenia are still on the decline. So, even though Skunk [a high cannabinoid content cannabis strain] has been around now for 10 years, there has been no upswing in schizophrenia. In fact, where people have looked, they haven't found any evidence linking cannabis use in a population and schizophrenia."[6]

In 2012, a report authored by Leweke et al was published with regard to psychosis and schizophrenia and in stark contrast to the official government assertions that cannabis causes schizophrenia, the study found instead that cannabidiol (CBD) enhances anandamide signaling and actually alleviates the psychotic symptoms of schizophrenia and that CBD was as effective as amisulpride, a standard antipsychotic.[7]

When Dr. Lester Grinspoon was the Associate Professor Emeritus of Psy-

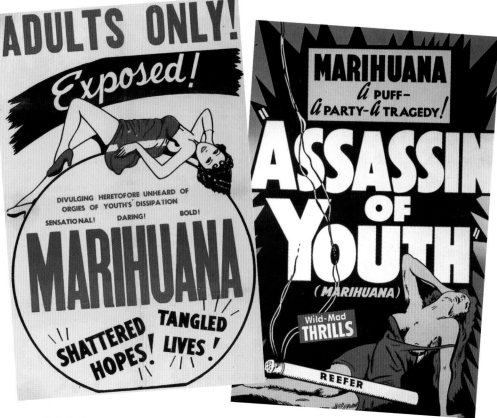

Pulp fiction.

chiatry at Harvard Medical School and senior psychiatrist at the Massachusetts Mental Health Center in Boston, he stated:

> "If the brain produces its own cannabinoid-like substances, it doesn't make much sense that it would produce a substance which is going to damage the brain.[8] Indeed, long before it was discovered that there are endogenous cannabinoids, the empirical evidence did not demonstrate that cannabis damaged the brain."

Another spurious argument put forward by those wishing to keep cannabis illegal is the "gateway" theory. The prohibitionists like to imply that cannabis consumers will go on to become users of hard drugs such as heroin and cocaine. This discredited theory is unsupported by any medical evidence; in fact,

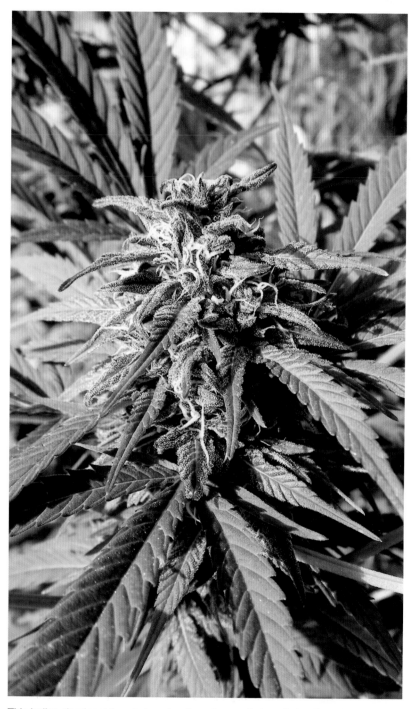

This indica-dominant female has developed a purple hue during flowering.

researchers have reported that they have found that the gateway theory argument can be better applied to alcohol and tobacco, as these are actually the first drugs that most people experience.[9] Cannabis has also been shown to be a useful medication in the treatment of alcoholism and drug addiction, and in medical trials it has been shown to reduce the user's cravings for cocaine. Research published in many peer-reviewed scientific journals indicates that the cannabis plant's addictive potential is less than that of caffeine.[10]

The idea that cannabis is a gateway drug is so erroneous that modern scientific journals rarely bother to publish work on the issue. It is a scientifically established fact that the majority of people who try cannabis do not progress to experimentation with harder drugs and in most cases they do not even go on to use cannabis regularly.[11]

The third argument put forward to justify cannabis prohibition is even more ridiculous, but nonetheless steadfastly repeated by politicians and prohibitionists alike. When asked about the possibility of legalization, they will claim that cannabis strains are now much stronger than they were in the past, and therefore present a health risk. New strains may well have more cannabinoid content, although many would argue that Thai sticks and Afghani indica strains were just as potent 20 years ago. Irrespective of this, cannabis is medically proven to be safe, regardless of its cannabinoid content. If the cannabis of today is more potent, then the only side effect is that users will become more stoned and more easily remedied by consuming less.

The only recorded side effect of any note is known as "cannabis hyperemesis" and, although non–life threatening, it produces unpleasant and debilitating symptoms in a very small number of people.[12] This rare and unusual syndrome is associated with chronic cannabis use and was recently reported in seven case reports of patients from Australia, with a further eight well-documented cases in the United States. It is estimated that there are approximately 750,000 people who regularly use cannabis in Australia and over 17,000,000 users in the U.S., so the occurrence is extremely uncommon.[13, 14] Cannabis hyperemesis is characterized by otherwise unexplained recurrent nausea and vomiting, compulsive bathing, abdominal pain and excessive thirst. Ceasing cannabis use results in complete symptomatic recovery. Abstaining totally from cannabis for 30 days before restarting consumption is a remedy for most sufferers, though this condition could be very serious for cancer patients if it struck during a course of cannabis oil treatment.

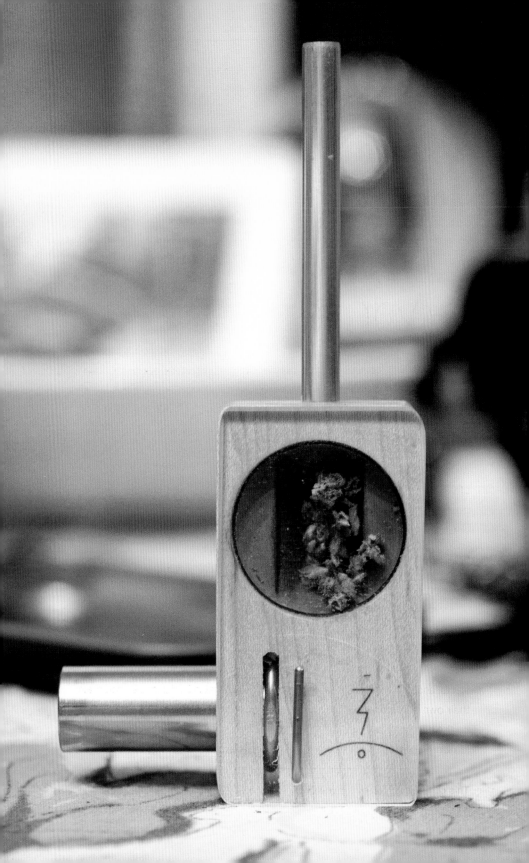

CHAPTER THREE

Administration

Cannabis is one of the safest and most effective medications known today, with the potential to treat a wide variety of medical conditions. By the early 19th century, the benefits of medicinal cannabis use had become widely acknowledged in the West, having been brought to France by Napoleon's army as they returned from Egypt, where cannabis was commonly used for its analgesic and sedative qualities.[1] Medical cannabis became universally accepted after extensive research by the Irish physician William O'Shaughnessy, who published a paper in 1843 entitled *On the Preparations of the Indian Hemp, or Gunjah*, which is noted for having introduced cannabis sativa to European and American medicine.[2] O'Shaughnessy experimented with alcoholic tinctures and found this to be an effective way of isolating the major psychoactive component found in cannabis, delta-9-tetrahydrocannabinol (THC).

From 1890 to 1937, Parke, Davis & Company (now part of the Pfizer Group of Companies) marketed many formulations of medicinal cannabis, including tinctures that were available by the pint or fluid ounce and cannabis tablets that could be bought by the gram.[3] It was also possible to purchase powdered extracts, and even pressed flowering tops (dried cannabis buds) for users to make their own preparations. All products and formulations were proudly advertised by the company as "originating from American home-grown cannabis." Pfizer is now one of the world's top pharmaceutical companies; in 2009 it made

....

This portable vaporizer is a great way to administer your medical cannabis.

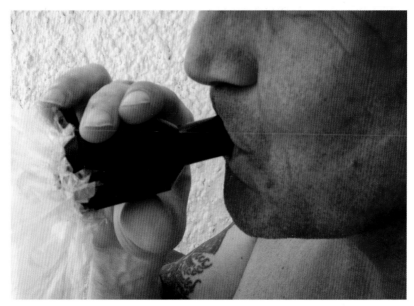

Mel Thomas inhaling pure CBD vapor from a vaporizer bag.

$50 billion profit in annual sales of prescription drugs, many of which replaced cannabis medications.[4]

Another major manufacturer of cannabis preparations and still a familiar name today is Eli Lilly & Co, who, from 1877 to 1935, manufactured and sold fluid, solid, and powdered extracts, all of which were stated to be manufactured from the flowering tops of the pistillate plants of cannabis sativa.[5] Merck and Squibb are also both well-known pharmaceutical manufacturing companies that in the past have sold and marketed cannabis preparations.[6] The two companies extensively advertised that they supplied dried flowering tops of the female cannabis plant. In addition, Merck was also a manufacturer and supplier of cannabis fluid extracts, tinctures, pills and cannabis oil made from infused tops.[7]

Alcohol-based tinctures are still used by pharmaceutical companies today; indeed, Sativex, a cannabinoid-based medicine, is basically a cannabis tincture spray. It has a cannabinoid profile of 51% THC and 49% CBD suspended in alcohol and is produced using organic cannabis, just like the tinctures made by Eli Lilly & Co over 150 years ago.[8]

A 2008 report by the Florida Medical Examiners Commission concluded that prescription medications easily exceed illegal drugs as a major cause of death.[9] An analysis of 168,900 autopsies conducted in Florida found that three times as many people were killed by pharmaceutical drugs than by cocaine, heroin and methamphetamines put together.[10] Cocaine was responsible for 843 deaths, heroin for 121, and methamphetamines for 25. Cannabis accounted for no deaths whatsoever. In contrast, 2,328 people were killed by opioid painkillers, including Vicodin and OxyContin, and 743 were killed by drugs containing benzodiazepine, including Valium and Xanax.[11]

In the U.S., over 40,000 people are killed annually by aspirin and painkillers.[12] According to *The American Journal of Medicine*, over 100,000 patients are hospitalized annually for non-steroidal anti-inflammatory drug (NSAID)–related gastrointestinal complications and at least 16,500 deaths occur each year among arthritis patients alone.[13] A report in *The New England Journal of Medicine* stated:

"It has been estimated conservatively that 16,500 NSAID-related deaths

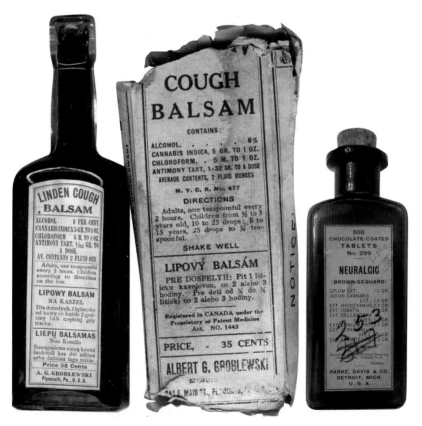

Surgeon W.B. O'Shaughnessy introduced cannabis into Western medicine in the 1840s.

occur among patients with rheumatoid arthritis or osteoarthritis every year in the United States.[14] This figure is similar to the number of deaths from AIDS and considerably greater than the number of deaths from multiple myeloma, asthma, cervical cancer or Hodgkin's disease. If deaths from gastrointestinal toxic effects from NSAID were tabulated separately in the National Vital Statistics reports, these effects would constitute the 15th most common cause of death in the United States. Yet these toxic effects remain mainly a 'silent epidemic,' with many physicians and most patients unaware of the magnitude of the problem. Furthermore the mortality statistics do not include deaths ascribed to the use of over-the-counter NSAIDS."

Medical Cannabis Today

The two main cannabis strains used for medical cannabis are the cannabis indica and cannabis sativa subspecies, which owing to their cannabinoid profiles both differ in their medicinal properties. Cannabis strains are available across the entire spectrum, from pure cannabis sativas to pure cannabis indicas and combinations which are known as hybrids. The resulting hybrid strains will grow and develop medicinal properties relative to the dominant genetics they inherit; for example, cannabis indica strains have more chlorophyll than cannabis sativa, and so grow and mature faster. Furthermore, cannabis indica-dominant plants can have a CBD/THC ratio four to five times that of cannabis sativa-dominant hybrids. Auto-flowering plants containing cannabis rudralis genetics are fine for medical use; just choose either an indica- or sativa-dominant hybrid depending on your particular needs. The effects of cannabis sativa are well known for inducing a THC cerebral high, hence they tend to be used medicinally during the daytime. As the effects of cannabis indicas are predominantly physical and sedative, they are best used for non-active times of the day, being particularly beneficial when used before sleeping. To determine the best strain for your condition it is important to understand the different effects of these two subspecies:

Cannabis indica-dominant strains tend to have a more sedative effect on the user and help to relieve stress and aid relaxation. These plants are recommended for pain relief when vaporized, and for cancer treatment in the form of an oil extraction. They can also help moderate nausea, stimulate the appetite, and reduce intraocular pressure. Most medical cannabis emanates from cannabis indica hybrids. A few examples of these hybrid strains include:

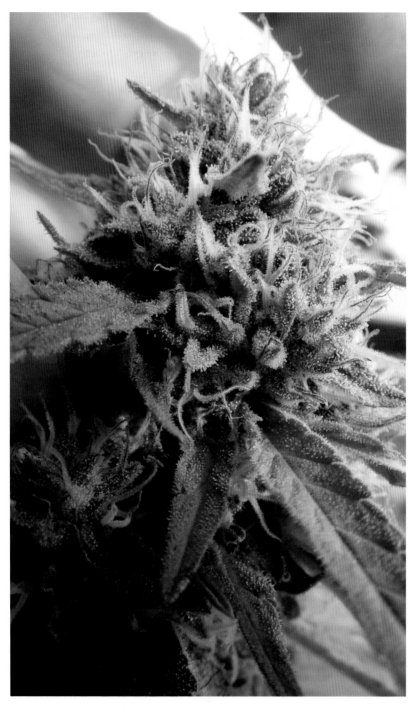

As the female flower approaches harvest, the white pistils turn brown.

OG Kush, Master Kush, Purple Kush, White Rhino, Blueberry, Grapefruit, Lemon Skunk and Northern Lights. Predominantly cannabis indica strains are recommended for treating anxiety, cancer, chronic pain, insomnia, muscle spasms and tremors, and for their effectiveness for appetite stimulation, increase in dopamine production, nausea reduction and sedative action.

Cannabis sativa-dominant strains are more energizing, enhance a feeling of well-being and stimulate the neurotransmitter serotonin, a type of chemical that helps relay signals from one area of the brain to another. Of the approximately 40 million brain cells we have, most are influenced either directly or indirectly by serotonin, which also acts on the central nervous system and, amongst other things, is responsible for mood and appetite regulation. Consumption of pure cannabis sativa strains can often induce paranoia attacks and irregular heartbeat, so hybrids also containing cannabis indica are preferred for medicinal use. These hybrids are useful for the antidepressant properties they possess, without inducing the paranoia associated with purebred cannabis sativa, but they rarely have any pain-blocking attributes, so cannabis indicas are preferred for use as analgesics.

The high THC content of many cannabis sativa hybrids is useful in treating any conditions where CBD content is not so useful, such as glaucoma and multiple sclerosis. Common cannabis sativa-dominant hybrids include Haze, Kali Mist, Jack Herer, Willy Nelson and Cheese. Cannabis sativa-dominant strains are recommended for use in treating depression, chronic fatigue syndrome, loss of appetite, cancer, migraines, nausea and as a daytime medication.

Treating Internal Cancers with Cannabis Oil

Providing the treatment is started early enough, the oral administration of cannabis oil benefits most patients diagnosed with cancer.

If you're a cancer patient beginning treatment with cannabis oil, it is recommended that you make some dietary changes and it is advisable to cut out red meat altogether. Use more hemp seed, oily fish and vegetables such as broccoli, spinach, corn or potatoes for your protein (see appendix I). Do not drink alcohol as this would be adding additional complications. It has been shown that regularly drinking around 3 units of alcohol a day (a large glass of wine) can increase the risk of mouth, throat, esophageal, breast and bowel cancers.

Rick Simpson, in his work, advises that patients should also take high doses of vitamin C daily. The authors have themselves been successfully treating cancer patients for over a decade using cannabis oil and whilst they

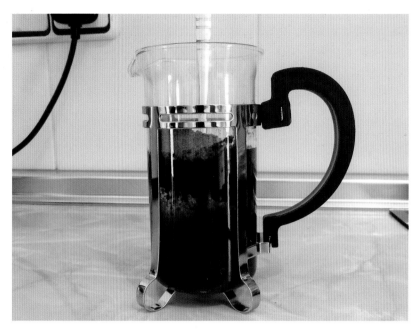

Bud Buddies 1:1 ratio CBD:THC cannabis oil as produced by the authors.

advise making a dietary change they don't agree with Simpson on this issue. The claim that vitamin C is useful in the treatment of cancer is largely attributable to Linus Pauling, PhD.[15] In 1976 and 1978, he and a Scottish surgeon, Ewan Cameron, reported that patients treated with high doses of vitamin C (10,000 milligrams per day) had survived three to four times longer than similar patients who did not receive vitamin C supplements.

Extensive studies have been carried out on Linus Pauling's claims that high-dose vitamin C prolonged the life of cancer patients, and these found that the claims were based on improper statistical analysis of data. Subsequent clinical trials found no benefit from his recommendations. Case reports also indicate that very high doses of vitamin C can cause kidney damage and interfere with the body's ability to absorb copper; therefore even if supplementary vitamin C is eventually found to have some use in fighting cancer, that role is not likely to be extensive. Vitamin C is a potent antioxidant that does help the body protect its cells, and there is no harm in taking up to 1000 milligrams daily as a supplement.[16] However, it won't cure cancer and may give you diarrhea, which will cause dehydration. If you do wish to increase your intake, it is far better to do this by consuming foods that are high in vitamin C content.

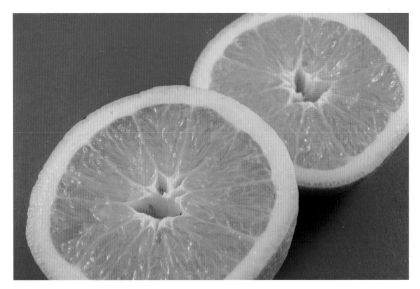

Adopting a healthy Mediterranean-style diet is proven to reduce cancer.

Other than these changes, all you require is the cannabis oil itself. Do not buy this from dealers on the black market as the purity will not be sufficiently high. Make a pure, high-quality oil yourself using a cannabis indica variety high in CBD content such as Skunk Haze (from the CBD Crew) and follow the techniques described in this book. One pound of dried cannabis flowers will produce around two ounces of high-grade cannabis oil, which is sufficient to treat even the most serious of cancers, if taken early enough.

Chemotherapy

Chemotherapy is the general term for pharmaceutical cancer-inhibiting drugs. There is conflicting advice given on whether cancer patients should use cannabis oil before or during chemotherapy. Recently, a team of researchers looking into why cancer cells are so resilient discovered that chemotherapy seriously damages healthy cells and subsequently triggers them to release a protein that sustains and fuels tumor growth, making the tumor highly resistant to future treatment.[17] Reporting their findings in the journal *Nature Medicine,* the scientists state that their findings were "completely unexpected." After extensive research, Dr. Peter Nelson and his team at the Fred Hutchinson Cancer Research Center in Seattle found that chemotherapy helps cancer to survive, grow faster, and resist treatment.[18]

The team was trying to explain why cancer is so resilient in the body, yet so easy to kill in the lab, and realized that the culprit is the interaction of chemotherapy and healthy cells surrounding the targeted tumors. When used on cancer, chemotherapy slows or stops the reproduction of rapidly dividing cells found in tumors, but it also damages the DNA of neighboring fibroblast cells, which normally help heal wounds. These cells then produce 30 times more than normal of a protein called WNT16B. This protein encouraged prostate tumors to grow and spread into surrounding tissue, as well as to resist chemotherapy. The team examined cancer cells from prostate, breast and ovarian cancer patients who had been treated with chemotherapy and found similar results. It is up to the patient to make an informed decision as to whether he or she wishes to undergo chemotherapy or not but certainly the earlier you start cannabis oil treatment the better.

Dosage (Cancer)

The general consensus is that cancer sufferers require a treatment course total of 2 ounces (56 grams) of cannabis oil, to be ingested over a three-month period for maximum effectiveness. The dose is gradually built up to 1 gram a day. After this, many survivors continue a maintenance dose to keep the cancer at bay; this varies between individuals and the severity of their illness, but averages at 100-200 milligrams daily. The oil produced using the techniques

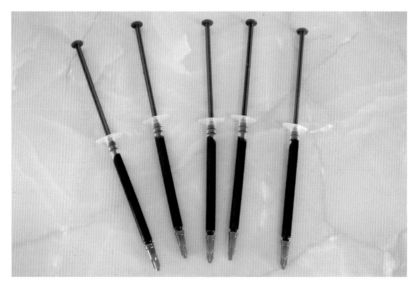

Bud Buddies 1:1 CBD:THC oil.

we describe will be extremely potent, so patients are advised to begin their treatment with very small doses starting off with dabs the size of a match head to be taken four times a day. For initial doses patients generally find that having the oil in a syringe enables them to easily squeeze the required amount onto their finger and then place this into the mouth.

The dose should be increased slowly every three to five days depending on the patient's tolerance, until they are able to take one gram daily. A set of digital scales accurate to a tenth of a gram are required to enable patients to accurately measure their consumption, however, it is not possible to overdose on cannabis oil and your body will not become dependent. Medically a patient has to be in remission for five years before being declared cancer-free, so once the course has been completed, it is recommended that you continue a maintenance dose of cannabis oil, the general consensus being between one tenth to one fifth of a gram per day.

General Administration of Cannabis

There are basically five methods of administering cannabis: inhalation (smoking), ingestion (eating), suppositories (anally), topically (creams) and also by intravenous injection (IV).

When choosing a route of administration it is important to exercise caution and build up your dose slowly. The side effects of over-consuming cannabinoids wear off quickly and will not have any detrimental long-term effects, but the immediate experience can be unpleasant for some individuals. The two most widely used routes of administration are inhalation and ingestion.

Smoking

Vaporizing or smoking cannabis is the preferred method for pain relief, as the effects are felt very quickly. When cannabinoids are drawn into the lungs, they rapidly enter the bloodstream, with the initial effects being felt within 20 seconds. First-time consumers who choose to try inhalation are advised to leave at least ten minutes between medications so they can gauge the effects. It is much easier to get the correct dosage when you inhale cannabis; as soon as you feel the effect you wish for, you should stop inhaling.

For most smokers, the preferred method is the traditional joint, which is simply made using cigarette papers rolled into a cigarette containing cannabis; it is not recommended that you include tobacco. When you smoke a joint, the

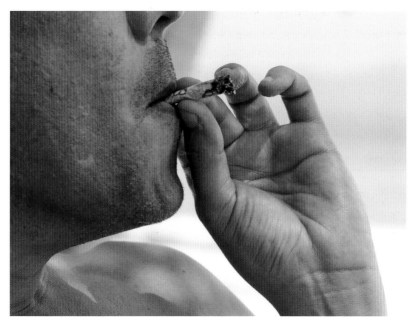

Consuming cannabis with tobacco is not recommended.

combustion occurring at the tip generates temperatures of around 1,112°F (600°C); when you draw (inhale) the temperature rises to around 1,652°F (900°C). These temperatures deliver the cannabinoids. However, the act of combustion also creates harmful gases such as benzene and toluene. There are conflicting arguments concerning the harmful effects of smoking cannabis. Some studies have indicated that smoking cannabis without tobacco is much less harmful than when they are consumed together, but other studies have concluded that even the smoking of cannabis without tobacco is damaging.

The results from one of the most comprehensive studies ever carried out on cannabis use and lung disorders was published in *The Journal of the American Medical Association*.[19] Researchers working on a long-term study of risk factors for cardiovascular disease (the Coronary Artery Risk Development in Young Adults or CARDIA study) tested the lung function of 5,115 young adults over the course of 20 years, starting in 1985 when they were aged between 18 and 30. Whilst tobacco smokers showed the expected decrease in lung function, the research found that cannabis smoke had unexpected and seemingly positive effects. Low to moderate users actually showed increased lung capacity compared to non-smokers on two tests. The first test, known as

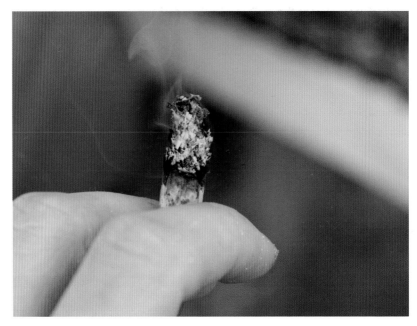

A pure cannabis joint containing no tobacco.

FEV1, is the amount of air someone breathes out in the first second after tak-ing the deepest possible breath; FVC is the second test and records the total volume of air exhaled after the deepest inhalation. Dr. Mark Pletcher, Associate Professor of Epidemiology and Biostatistics at the University of California, San Francisco and the lead author of the study, stated:

"FEV1 and FVC both actually increased with moderate and occasional use of marijuana. That was a bit of a surprise, there are clearly adverse effects from tobacco use and marijuana smoke has a lot of the same constituents as tobacco smoke does so we thought it might have some of the same harmful effects. It's a weird effect to see and we couldn't make it go away."[20]

Results indicate that smoking cannabis, even regularly and heavily, does not lead to lung cancer. Donald Tashkin of the University of California at Los Angeles, a pulmonologist who has studied cannabis for 30 years, states:

"We hypothesized that there would be a positive association between mar-ijuana use and lung cancer, and that the association would be more positive with heavier use. What we found instead was no association at all, and even a suggestion of some protective effect."[21]

Water-cooled pipes or bongs can also be used for inhalation, and many medical users choose this method. Smaller hand held pipes can also be used, and as long as you choose a small bowl model designed specifically for cannabis, the fumes inhaled when smoking will not be unnecessarily hot. Pipes and bongs are readily available for purchase online if you do not have a suitable store nearby. It should be remembered that smoking is not a very efficient method of delivering your medication, as the act of combustion destroys over 50% of the cannabinoids.

Vaporizers

A much more efficient and precise method of inhalation is a specially designed vaporizer. These units don't actually burn the cannabis material, but instead gently heat to set temperatures that release the cannabinoids as a mild vapor that can be inhaled.

A vaporizer does not use combustion, so none of the cannabinoids are consumed by flame, making a vaporizer very economical. With a quality vaporizer you are receiving 100% of the cannabinoids from your herbal cannabis, as opposed to losing over half of the cannabinoids through combustion when smoking.

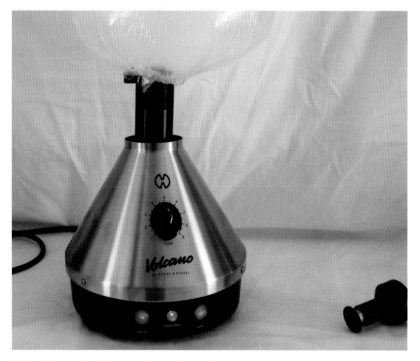

Volcano vaporizer. The vapor is collected in the bag for inhaling.

Vaporizers are usually portable and can be carried with you, with some being small enough to place in your pocket. The non-portable types are larger, and ideally you should purchase one that includes a variable temperature function that gives more precise delivery of the cannabinoids. The ability to choose the temperature at which you vaporize will allow you to administer the cannabinoids you wish, and, whether your desire is to medicate or get high, this essential facility gives you total control. It is the higher temperatures involved in smoking that are responsible for the production of carcinogenic hydrocarbons, and these are almost completely eliminated by the use of a quality vaporizer, as the lack of combustion suppresses the formulation of the health-damaging compounds. In 2007, a study of vaporization conducted at the San Francisco General Hospital concluded:

"Vaporization is a safe and effective cannabinoid delivery mode for patients who desire the rapid onset of action associated with inhalation while avoiding the respiratory risks of smoking, as they significantly reduced the intake of gaseous combustion toxins, including carbon monoxide."[22]

The vaporizer used by the 18 participants in the study was a Volcano Vaporizer, manufactured by Storz & Bickel, which was chosen for its reliability, efficiency and its accurate temperature control. Many Volcano owners find that its advantages more than compensate for its lack of portability. The Volcano is known as a "bag type" vaporizer, and works by generating heat via a thermostatically controlled heating element. When the desired temperature is reached, the operator activates a fan that blows the hot air through the chamber containing the cannabis. The air passing through the ground cannabis in the chamber is collected in a plastic bag, and then inhaled via a mouthpiece attachment. As well as efficiently vaporizing ground and dried cannabis buds, a good quality vaporizer should also be capable of vaporizing cannabis oil and hashish.

Researchers reported that vaporization resulted in higher plasma concentrations of THC compared to smoked cannabis for up to 60 minutes following inhalation. Investigators also reported that subjects self-titrated their intake of cannabis vapor, taking smaller and less frequent puffs when exposed to stronger cannabis. On average, the Volcano vaporizer exposed subjects to 54% of the applied dose of THC. Previous studies have shown that as much as 80% of the THC burned in cigarettes or water pipes is lost in slipstream smoke.

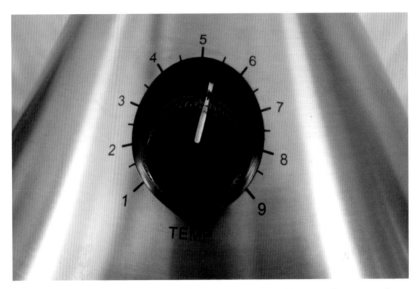

Variable heat settings allow you to select which cannabinoid you prefer to vaporize.

To get the best from your vaporizer, you have to be aware of the cannabinoid profile of the cannabis you are vaporizing, as you will only obtain high levels of CBD if it is actually present. If you wish mainly to experience the effects of THC, do not set your temperature control above 320°F (160°C). After a couple of bags, you can increase the temperature to allow the release of CBD or you may wish to save the already vaporized cannabis for later use. To get the best out of your vaporizer, you should experiment; you may find that vaporizing THC during the day and re-vaporizing the same cannabis at a higher temperature in the evening is a good regimen. As an alternative to re-vaporizing you may prefer to use the remaining cannabinoids in an edible form or cannabis preparation.

CANNABINOID RECOMMENDED TEMPERATURES
THC 284-320°F (140-160°C)
CBD 320-356°F (160-180°C)
CBN 365°F (185°C)
CBC 428°F (220°C)

Temperatures in excess of 446°F (230°C) will produce benzene and other harmful chemicals.

The cannabis plant also produces terpenoid essential oils, which are responsible for its distinctive aromas and tastes and also have beneficial medicinal properties. Like the cannabinoids, they evaporate at set temperatures.

TERPENOID PROPERTIES TEMP

ß-caryophyllene Anti-inflammatory 248°F (120°C)

a-pinene Bronchodilator stimulant 312°F (156°C)

ß-myrcene Analgesic & Anti-inflammatory 330°F (166°C)

d-limonene Antidepressant 350°F (177°C)

linalool Sedative 388°F (198°C)

pulegone Sedative 435°F (224°C)

The inhalation of cannabinoid oils in this fashion is referred to as "dabbing," and the amount of oil (dab) used per dose will usually vary between 0.1 and 0.8 of a gram.

Ingestion

There are many edible preparations of cannabis. Patients who are ingesting or eating cannabis for the first time should be cautious as the effects can take between 30 minutes to three hours to be felt, depending on the preparation and the metabolism of the individual. With such a wide variance it's possible to inadvertently take an additional dose before the full effects of the initial dose have been felt.

It is important when ingesting cannabis to know the cannabinoid content of the preparation being consumed. This is much easier if you are making the edibles yourself, as you have complete control over the potency and strength. If you live in an area where medical cannabis is legal and you obtain your cannabis edibles and preparations from a dispensary, the cannabinoid content should be clearly displayed on the product. When ingesting cannabis, it is far more effective to consume your necessary dose on an empty stomach.

Capsules

These are useful for ease of administration and monitoring dose, so many patients choose to encapsulate their cannabinoid oil concentrate. Empty 500-milligram capsules made from plant starch are available online. The capsules come in two halves and you fill one half with oil at your required dosage, then close the cap with the other half.

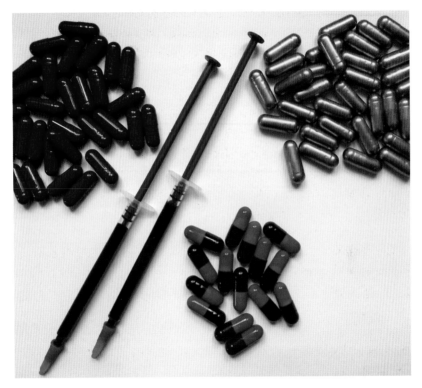

1:1 CBD:THC cannabis oil preparations.

Cannabis Tinctures (Alcohol)

These are an excellent way to utilize the plant's medicinal ingredients, and a good alternative to smoking. Tinctures are easy to make and involve soaking your dried cannabis buds in ethanol or ethyl alcohol. The proof listed on commercial alcohol refers to the percentage of ethanol that the drink contains. The proof is twice the percentage (purity), so 70 proof means that the mixture contains 35% ethanol. The higher the alcohol content, the better the extraction. High-proof spirits such as Everclear 95% pure grain alcohol can be difficult to obtain, but if you have access to these products, they are ideal to use.

When you are making a tincture, the cannabis used must be absolutely dry and decarboxylated by gently heating in an oven at 110°C (230°F) to activate the cannabinoids. The process of heating converts the cannabinoid acids such as THCA into THC. It is advisable to chop but not finely grind the material before use. The cannabis should be soaked from between one and 10 days, with around seven days being adequate. The recommended minimum effective ratio

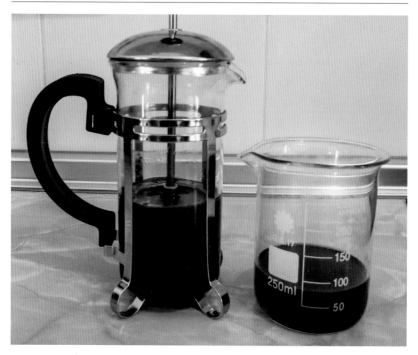

Cannabis oil can be easily made at home using kitchen equipment.

to use is one gram of bud per 35 milliliters (one fluid ounce) of alcohol, with up to eight grams per 35 milliliters used for those preferring a stronger tincture. Place the solution into a sealed jar that you can periodically shake to assist in the process. Throughout the soaking period use only enough ethanol to cover the plant material. To make what is known as a "cold extraction", place the jar in the freezer compartment of your refrigerator and remove periodically to shake the container. This cold extraction can be completed in around four days, but is not necessary for good results.

Once the soaking process has finished, strain the solution, and then further purify it by filtering through a coffee filter. Store the tincture in a cool dark place, preferably in a bottle with a dropper. Because of the varying strengths of tinctures, patients should experiment with small doses until the desired effect is achieved. Administer under the tongue using the dropper.

You can further concentrate the tincture by reducing the volume of the alcohol by evaporation; the more alcohol you evaporate the more potent the tincture will be. Evaporate too much though, and you will have an oil and not a tincture!

Cannabis Tincture (Glycerin)

For those who prefer not to use alcohol, food-grade glycerin is an alternative solvent. Using ½ gallon (64 fluid ounces) of food-grade glycerin will be sufficient to process three ounces (84 grams) of quality cannabis buds. Again, the more cannabis you add, the more potent and stronger it will be. Unlike the "cold tincture" method with the alcohol tincture, a glycerin tincture requires some heat to assist the absorption of the cannabinoids. The plant material should be finely ground and placed into a crock pot (slow cooker) on the lowest setting, and left to heat for at least 12 hours with the lid on. Ensure the setting is low enough not to burn the mixture. After the heating process allow the mixture to cool and strain as before.

Suppositories

The most common form of suppository is the rectal suppository, a very effective method of administration for the delivery of cannabinoids. Suppositories are designed to dissolve or melt and this allows the active ingredients (in this case cannabinoids) to enter the bloodstream via the blood vessels lining the rectum. There are many advantages to this method of administration:

- Works faster than when taken orally.
- Avoids the production of the very psychoactive 11-Hydroxy-THC.
- Requires a lower dose due to increased bioavailability.
- Very effective for delivering cannabinoids to people who cannot take them orally due to nausea and vomiting.
- The effects are longer lasting.

Suppositories are very easy to make. Add half a gram of oil to three grams of natural cocoa butter, slowly melt, and mix thoroughly. Professional suppository molds are available online, or alternatively you can create a simple mold by wrapping tin foil round your little finger. If you have made capsules for oral application, these can also be used as a suppository. However, some people may find that they need to apply a small amount of lubricant to aid insertion.

Studies indicate that using THC-HS suppositories for rectal administration offers around twice the bioavailability of oral administration.[23] Converting THC into the ester THC-HS makes it water soluble, improving uptake and bioavailability. However, the esterfication of cannabinoids is beyond the scope of this book.

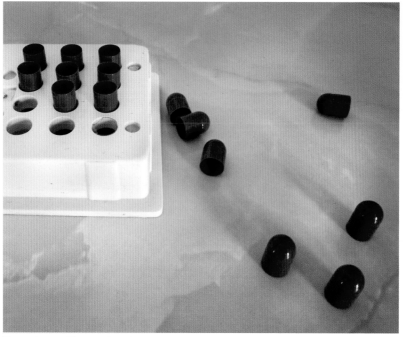

Preparing to fill capsules with cannabis oil.

From our own studies, we have found that using half-gram oil capsules as suppositories is twice as effective as when they are taken orally. To put this into context, it means that you are using the oil you have more efficiently and require less.

Cannabis Cream for Topical Application

Cannabis cream is recommended to help with arthritis and has also been successful for some psoriasis sufferers. To convert cannabis oil into a cream, simply melt cocoa butter or beeswax and mix thoroughly with the oil. Add 50 milliliters of oil to 100 grams of cocoa butter or beeswax.

Cannabis oil can also be applied directly to the skin without the need to make a cream preparation and this is the recommended method for treating skin cancer, burns and warts.

Intravenous (IV)

In 1968 Henderson and Pugsley first described the syndrome of emesis, myalgia and hypotension following the IV injection of broth derived from boiled

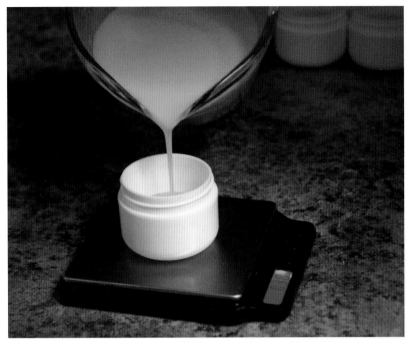

Cannabis-based creams can offer relief for many skin conditions.

cannabis that was then strained through cotton cloth.[24] The syndrome has at least 25 known cases in the English language literature, all prior to 1983. Symptoms include myalgia, nausea and vomiting, diarrhea, abdominal pain and weakness. In at least seven cases, cotton was used to strain the broth before injecting and it is noteworthy that "cotton fever" has been reported following the IV use of heroin reclaimed from previously used cotton filters and also consists of emesis, myalgia and fever. Thus, it partially resembles the IV marijuana syndrome. All known patients recovered with normal care, with an average hospital stay of 9 days.

The psychoactive constituents of cannabis are terpenoids. These are not water soluble and thus not suitable for a broth-type preparation for injection with any efficacy. A laboratory setting for injection of cannabinoids would use a lipid soluble intravenous emulsion vehicle such as soy lecithin for injection. Additionally, the cannabinoids would need to be decarboxylated in order to cross the blood-brain barrier. [25]

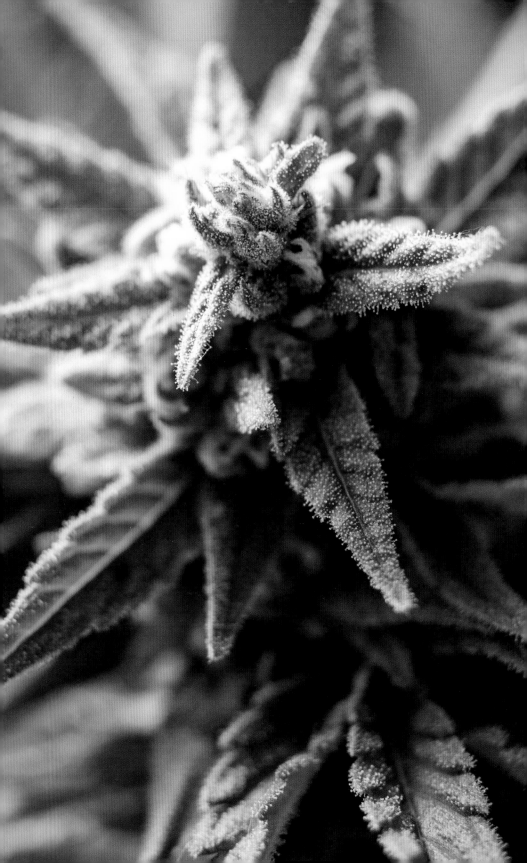

CHAPTER FOUR

Cannabis Cures

Studies carried out in California to determine why patients used cannabis for medicinal purposes reported that it relieved pain, muscle spasms, headaches, anxiety, nausea, vomiting, depression, cramps, panic attacks, diarrhea and itching.

Others reported that cannabis improved sleep, relaxation, appetite, concentration and energy. Many patients use it to prevent side effects from medication or to treat anger issues, involuntary muscle movements and seizures whilst others used it as a substitute for prescription drugs and alcohol. It can be argued that recreational cannabis use is also of medical benefit in that it relieves stress and thereby acts as a preventative treatment for many stress-related conditions.

If you are diagnosed with any of the conditions that can be treated with cannabis, you are advised to consult with your physician before you begin self-medicating. However, in some countries, such as the U.K., a doctor has a duty to report any illegal drug use that may impair a patient's ability to drive, so such a confession could have consequences.

Many medical practitioners are becoming aware of the benefits of cannabis medication and most will have no objection to you using it alongside any treatment you may be receiving.

Cannabinoid crystals are evident even on the plant's smallest buds. These crystals are commonly known as trichomes. They also appear here on the plant's sugar leaves.

Case History: Corrie Yelland

Corrie Yelland is a remarkable and determined lady who refused serious radiation treatment and against all odds cured her terminal cancer using only cannabis oil.[1] In May of 2007 she suffered a heart attack and subsequently had a double heart bypass. As a result of the heart surgery she suffered with chronic debilitating pain from a maligned sternum and post sternotomy neuralgia/syndrome. She was constantly in pain and ingesting large amounts of various painkillers, and at night, even after taking sleeping pills, she would wake in agony within two hours of falling asleep.

In July of 2011, already coping with two spots of skin cancer on her collarbone, she was stunned to be diagnosed with anal canal cancer. Following two surgeries, the doctors told her that they could not remove all of the cancer and she would have to endure a regime of radiation treatments. She was informed that this was the worst area of the body to radiate as the radiation beam would hit both her coccyx and pubic bone potentially causing permanent damage. Additionally, she would suffer second and third degree burns vaginally and rectally, and there was a good possibility both her vagina and rectum would fuse shut from the burns and subsequent scarring.

Refusing to accept this was her only option, Corrie began to research alternatives and discovered information regarding the benefits of cannabis oil. She began a course of treatment soon after. As well as ingesting the cannabis oil, she topically applied it to the skin cancer on her collarbone. Within 48 hours, there were visible changes to the skin cancer. In just over a week, the two spots were completely gone. Elated, she continued ingesting the oil in the hope it would work on the other cancer attacking her body. Two weeks into her treatment regime the pain in her sternum, as well as the nerve pain, had become almost non-existent. Before using cannabis, Corrie typically took 10-15 Tylenol 3 per day, along with other drugs, which she managed to reduce to half a Tylenol 3 per day once treatment had began.

Corrie had met a woman from Texas diagnosed at the same time as her with the identical cancer. They gave each other support and felt fortunate to have found each other as they were identical in many respects: they were the same age, had gone through the same diagnostic procedure, were at the same stage of the cancer and both had radiation recommended as treatment. The Texan lady chose to have the radiation. Sadly she died in March 2012 as a result of infection from radiation burns. She left behind a husband and 12-

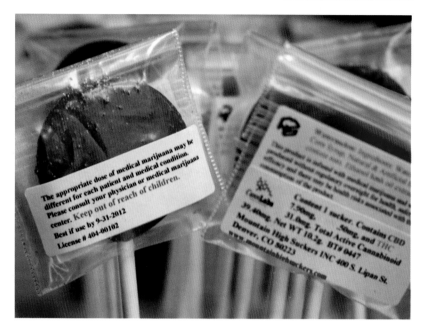

Medical marijuana is now available in many U.S. states.

year-old daughter.

Corrie continued ingesting the oil on a daily basis, slowly increasing the amount she was taking. She also began filling gelatin capsules with a mixture of the cannabis oil and olive oil and inserting them rectally. On September 20, 2012, she saw her specialist/surgeon again and heard the news she had only dared to hope for. "It's gone! I can't find anything at all. If it wasn't for the scar tissue I would never have known you had ever had cancer." She received confirmation that the cancer was confirmed to be 100% clear. You can read more of this remarkable story and view her medical notes, et cetera at the authors' website: www.cannabiscure.info/files/corrie.htm.

Conditions That Cannabis Can Assist With Include:

Alcohol and Opiate Abuse

Cannabis can ease both the physical and psychological effects associated with withdrawal from both of these addictive substances. No clinical trials concerning the efficacy of cannabis as a substitute for alcohol are available, apart from the work of Tod Mikuriya in 1970, who describes patients using cannabis to successfully discontinue abusing alcohol.[2] (*Cannabis as a Pharmacological*

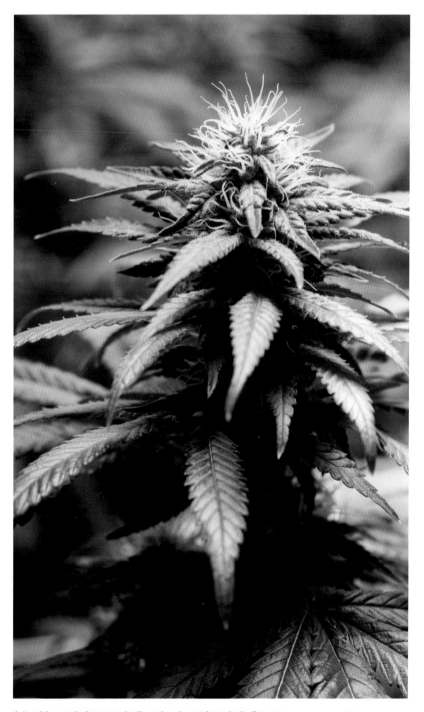

A healthy and vigorous indica-dominant female in flower.

Harm Reducer 1997–unpublished). Tod Hiro Mikuriya was a psychiatrist and an advocate for the legalization of the use of cannabis for medical purposes, and, quite fittingly, he is regarded as the grandfather of the medical cannabis movement in the United States.

Cannabis was listed as a treatment for delirium tremens in medical texts of the 1800s.[3] There are also 19th-Century references to the use of cannabis as a substitute for opiates. These were among the first documented uses of medical cannabis by European physicians.

It is apparent from reading the old medical texts that many of the new cannabis preparations and methods of administration around today are not new discoveries. They are, for the most part, just rediscoveries.

The U.S. Center for Disease Control and Prevention (CDC) reports that more than 80,000[4] annual deaths are attributed to alcohol use alone. Untreated and severe alcohol withdrawal can kill you, mainly due to seizures. Fortunately, these fatalities are almost completely preventable if people are properly weaned off alcohol using gradually decreasing amounts of alcohol itself or medication. In contrast, the CDC does not even have a category for deaths caused by the use of cannabis because there have never been any.

Alzheimer's Disease

Alzheimer's disease is the leading cause of dementia amongst the elderly, and with the ever-increasing population, cases of Alzheimer's disease are expected to triple over the next 50 years.[5] Investigation shows that cannabis can prevent the formation of deposits in the brain associated with this degenerative disease. Researchers at the Scripps Research Institute in California found that the active component of cannabis, Delta9-tetrahydrocannabinol (THC) inhibits the enzyme acetylcholinesterase (AChE) as well as prevents AChE-induced amyloid beta-peptide (Abeta) accumulation, the key indicator of Alzheimer's disease.[6] There is also research concluding that amongst the other cannabis compounds, cannabidiol (CBD), which has no psychotropic effect, may represent a very promising agent with the highest prospect for therapeutic use in Alzheimer's patients, many of whom would find that the effect of THC alone could actually add to the confusion they experience.

Whilst THC is recognized as an important compound in the treatment of dementia, it needs to be administered with a corresponding or even higher value of CBD, which research has shown will lessen the psychotropic effect of

THC on the elderly patient. This can easily be achieved by careful selection of the cannabis strain used for medication and high CBD content cannabis strains are recommended for use in the treatment of dementia patients. There are pharmaceutical medicines that can treat the symptoms of Alzheimer's, but there is no cure. Some medicines will keep memory loss and other symptoms from progressing but this is a short-term solution. Compared to drugs currently prescribed for the treatment of Alzheimer's disease, THC in particular has been shown to be a considerably superior inhibitor of Abeta accumulation.

Amyotrophic Lateral Sclerosis (ALS)

ALS, also known as Lou Gehrig's disease, is characterized by the death of motor neurons leading to loss of limb control, breathing, swallowing, speech and widespread cellular dysfunction.[7] The condition refers to a disease of the nerve cells in the brain and spinal cord that control voluntary muscle movement. This is a fatal, degenerative disease marked by progressive muscle weakness and atrophy. Research has shown that cannabis may help ALS patients by relieving pain, spasticity, drooling and appetite loss. In scientific studies it has been shown that THC, along with other cannabinoids, can benefit laboratory mice specifically bred with ALS. This mounting evidence of cannabinoids halting the progression of the condition has started to change the attitudes of doctors, and prominent researchers have recently called for ALS clinical trials with cannabinoids on humans.

Case History: Cathy Jordan[8]

Cathy Jordan was diagnosed with ALS in 1986 and given 3-5 years to live by her neurologist. Cathy began using cannabis to treat her ALS in the late 1980s. Nearly 3 decades later she is still alive and coping with ALS. Initially, doctors wouldn't accept that cannabis could be responsible for Cathy's survival and informed her that smoking anything would impair her lung function. Cathy asked her doctors if they would take a drug if it was neuroprotective, an antioxidant and anti-inflammatory. They replied that they would and asked her if she knew one, she informed them she did and it was cannabis. Cathy has said, "There are ALS patients' associations that fight for the right of patients to die with dignity. But what about my right to life? Keeping my medicine illegal removes my right to life."

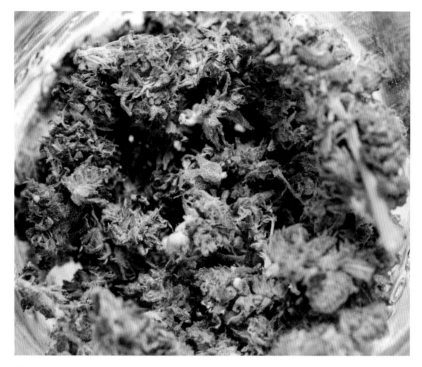

Dried and chopped cannabis bud ready for use.

Anorexia Nervosa

The prescription drug Olanzapine has been shown to be effective in treating certain aspects of this condition as it increases appetite, causes the body to store fat and helps to raise body mass index. However, the drug can have serious side effects including hives, difficulty breathing, swelling of the face, lips, tongue, or throat, high blood sugar, numbness or weakness, confusion, problems with vision, speech, or balance, fever, chills, body aches, flu-like symptoms, sores in the mouth and throat, swelling in the hands or feet and many other complications.[9] Cannabis has none of these side effects and can increase appetite and ease anxiety.[10] Dr. Elliot Berry, a consultant to the World Health Organization, has conducted a trial using cannabis oil to treat this eating disorder. Early results show that cannabinoids stimulate a chemical in the brain that effectively boosts appetite. In another unrelated trial it was reported that after 21 days of inpatient cannabis smoking, both body weight gain and caloric consumption were higher in casual and heavy users than in the control subjects who did not use cannabis.[11, 12, 13]

Arthritis (Rheumatoid or Osteoarthritis)

Rheumatoid arthritis is caused by a malfunction of the immune system. Instead of fighting bacteria or viruses, the body attacks the synovial membranes, which facilitate the movement of joints, eventually destroying cartilage and eroding bones. This manifests as a painful and debilitating inflammation of one or more joints. A joint is the area where two bones contact. When the body metabolizes THC it generates chemicals that include at least one that is an anti-inflammatory, THC also achieves relief from the pain associated with the condition.[14] Cannabidiol (CBD) is also useful in the treatment of arthritis and has been found to minimize destruction of the joints in laboratory rats and mice. Cannabis is beneficial not only when smoked by patients who seek relief from the symptoms, but it also works extremely well when applied topically as a cream.

Asthma

Cannabis use has been shown to ease asthma attacks in patients. Asthma is the shortness of breath and wheezing caused by spasms of the bronchial tubes, overproduction of mucus and swelling of the mucous membranes; it kills more than 4,000 U.S. citizens each year. Clinical research shows that THC acts as a bronchial dilator, clearing blocked air passageways and allowing free breathing. *The New England Journal of Medicine* published a 1973 study that claimed that, "Marihuana smoke, unlike cigarette smoke, causes broncho-dilation rather than broncho-constriction [narrowing of the air passages] and, unlike opiates, does not cause central respiratory depression."[15] Cannabis smoke at 2.6% THC content causes a fall of 38% in airway resistance and an increase of 44% in airway conductivity.[16] However, it is recommended that asthma sufferers use a vaporizer to relieve their symptoms rather than any other method of delivery.

Attention Deficit Hyperactivity Disorder (ADHD)

ADHD is one of the most common psychiatric disorders of childhood, and is characterized by persistent impairments in attention and concentration with the associated symptoms of impulsivity and hyperactivity.

Over 6.4 million children in the U.S. have been diagnosed with ADHD, and two thirds of those are currently taking drugs to control ADHD, fueling a $9-billion-a-year industry.[17] Although ADHD is most commonly treated with amphetamine-derived formulations, pure methamphetamine is actually approved by the FDA for the treatment of ADHD–they just prefer to call it Desoxyn (methamphetamine hydrochloride).[18] There is also growing concern about the use of Ritalin, the most widely prescribed drug for ADHD, and many parents and professionals are worried about side effects, including damage to the cardiovascular and nervous systems. A lack of dopamine is believed to be one of the primary underlying factors in ADHD.[19] This is the reason why stimulants are such an effective and commonly prescribed treatment, as stimulants mainly act to increase dopamine levels. Dysfunction of the dopamine (DA) system explains some of the clinical manifestations of attention-deficit/hyperactivity disorder (ADHD) and it is thought that the body releases its own natural cannabinoids as a protective response to the onset of ADHD-related symptoms. This would explain why ADHD sufferers gain relief from cannabis use.

Atherosclerosis

Atherosclerosis (also known as arteriosclerotic vascular disease or ASVD) is a condition in which an artery wall thickens as a result of the accumulation of fatty materials such as cholesterol. It is commonly referred to as a hardening or furring of the arteries, but is a disease where cholesterol deposits form on the inner surfaces of the arteries, obstructing blood flow. Cannabinoids, acting via both CB2 and CB1 receptor modulation, have an important role in immune system regulation. Because inflammation plays a key role in atherogenesis, cannabinoids can potentially affect atherogenesis via modulation of the immune system. In a pioneering study by Steffens et al, oral administration of low-dose THC (1 milligram per kilogram/day) was shown to inhibit progression of atherosclerotic lesions in the aortic root and abdominal aorta via activation of CB2 receptors on these cells.[20]

Autism

Autism Spectrum Disorder (ASD) is a developmental disorder that appears within the first 3 years of life and mainly affects communication and social skills. The cause of the disorder is not known but is linked to abnormal brain chemistry. Pharmaceutical medications are available to deal with the behavioral consequences of the disorder, but not the disorder itself. These pharmaceuticals have a host of serious side effects that include permanent tics (involuntary muscle movement) and diabetes, as well as being highly toxic chemicals. In 2000 researchers at the University of California at Irvine discovered that because of the interaction between the cannabinoids in the cannabis plant and the body's own natural endocannabinoid system it could be used to treat autism along with Parkinson's disease and schizophrenia.[21] Cannabinoids not only regulate emotion and focus but also serve as a neuroprotective preventing the further degradation of brain cells. Moderating an autistic person's mood consistently is best achieved with an oral dose of cannabis that can be adjusted according to need.

Case History: Marie Myung-Ok Lee[22]

Marie is a novelist who teaches at Columbia University and writes for *Slate, Salon, The New York Times,* and *The Guardian.* Marie has been treating her autistic son with legally acquired medical cannabis for several years. It has helped calm her son's gastrointestinal pain and decrease his associated violent behavior. Cannabis has allowed them to forego the use of pharmaceutical psychotropic drugs that were used to control aggressive outbursts, but were totally ineffective at alleviating his pain. Marie has written several essays regarding cannabis and autism and these can be found online. She states that, "In our case, I would call our experiment a qualified success. Not because cannabis has cured J, who's now 11, or anything near it. But it's alleviated some of his severest symptoms so that he, my husband and I can actually enjoy each other, rather than being held hostage by his autism in a house full of screams, destruction and three very unhappy people."

Bipolar Disorder

This is a psychiatric disorder characterized by extreme mood swings, ranging between episodes of acute euphoria, mania and severe depression. Cannabis is extremely beneficial in treating this condition (see Depression). Bipolar disorder is conventionally treated with lithium salts and anticonvulsant drugs, which can have serious side effects. Many sufferers report that cannabis is more effective than conventional anti-manic medication and can relieve the side effects associated with lithium use. Reports from the Zucker Hillside Hospital in New York show that patients with bipolar I (BD I) disorder who regularly used cannabis performed better on tests of attention, processing speed and working memory than other BD I patients.[23]

Cancer

Referred to medically as a malignant neoplasm, cancer is a broad group of various diseases, all involving unregulated cell growth. High concentrations of CBD found in cannabis oil have been shown to block the activity of a gene called Id-1, which is believed to be responsible for the aggressive spread of cancer cells away from the original tumor site (a process called metastasis). Research has shown that CBD can also reverse aggressive human brain cancers; it appears to have a similar effect on breast cancer cells, and is also highly effective in the treatment of lung cancer. A study by Complutense University of Madrid discovered that THC also has anticancer effects when treating brain tumors.[24] They found that the chemicals in cannabis promote the death of cancer cells by causing them to feed upon themselves in a process called autophagy.

Conventional medical practice uses surgery, highly toxic antineoplastic drugs, and/or the destruction of body tissue by radiation, which is energy directed at the tumor. It can range from what we think of as light photons to particles like electrons or even something as large as a carbon ion. Chemotherapy is classed as drug treatment and these are the main tools for treating cancer. Surgery is effective if carried out early enough, but chemotherapy is also commonly employed to treat patients and studies have raised serious questions about its efficacy–in particular the role it plays in hastening and even causing the death of late-stage cancer sufferers. One study carried out following patient outcome and deaths looked at the cases of 600 cancer sufferers who had passed on within 30 days of treatment.[25] The study found that approximately one in four of such deaths had either occurred far more rapidly, or been caused by chemotherapy. The study also revealed that two out of five patients had suffered significant poisoning from the treatment.

Moreover, a team of researchers studying cancer cell resilience discovered that chemotherapy seriously damages healthy cells and triggers them to release a protein that sustains and fuels tumor growth. Reporting their findings in *Nature Medicine*, the scientists reported that the results were completely unexpected and showed there was significant DNA damage from chemotherapy, using tissue derived from men with prostate cancer.[26] Furthermore, the tumors became highly resistant to future treatment. If you have recurring cancerous tumors, there is no effective conventional cure.

Studies published in *The Lancet* reported that use of the pharmaceutical drug Tamoxifen reduced the breast cancer death rate by one third.[27] The National Cancer Institute's breast cancer prevention trial stated that there was a 49% decrease in the incidence of this cancer in women who took it for five years.[28] However, when we examined the figures, we discovered that the risk of developing breast cancer without using the drug is only 1.3% and its use caused a reduction to 0.68%. That represents a 49% difference between these two reported numbers, but just a little over half of 1% difference (0.62%) in real terms. This is how the statistics are manipulated in favor of toxic pharmaceutical drugs.

Tamoxifen is a controversial synthetic hormone also sold in England as Nolvadex.[29] This toxic drug earns an estimated $500 million a year for the pharmaceutical companies; it's sold to women after breast surgery to prevent cancer from spreading to the other breast. *Science News* of March 4, 1989 reported slight benefits (9% in one study, 6% in another) but a Swedish trial indicated a 400% increased risk of endometrial cancer for those who took Tamoxifen over a 5-year period.[30, 31] Current guidelines for Tamoxifen recommend that patients take the drug for 5 years. The ATLAS study suggests that taking Tamoxifen for 10 years greatly increases a woman's survival rate from estrogen-positive breast cancers.[32] The ATLAS study was sponsored by none other than the drug manufacturer AstraZeneca that currently markets and manufactures Nolvadex, a brand-name version of the drug Tamoxifen. By doubling the number of years women take Tamoxifen, AstraZeneca doubles its profit! Tamoxifen is known to cause cancer of the uterus, ovaries and gastrointestinal tract and is shown to cause liver cancer. In 1996, a division of the World Health Organization declared Tamoxifen a Group I carcinogen for the uterus.[33] R. J. Kedar of King's College School of Medicine and Dentistry in London studied 61 women in a Tamoxifen trial and said: "Our study detected endometrial abnormalities at various times from the first tablet of Tamoxifen."[34] The endometrium appeared abnormally thick in 24 of these women (39%) and 10 of these underwent potentially precancerous changes. Other permanent damage includes osteoporosis, retina damage, optic nerve damage and cataracts. The half percent reduction in breast cancer rates is insignificant compared to the increased incidence of other cancers and diseases.

The medical use of cannabis causes none of these life-threatening complications. A team of researchers at the California Pacific Medical Center Research Institute who have been researching the benefits of CBD have concluded that it can provide a nontoxic alternative to chemotherapy for cancer treatments.[35] Dr Sean McAllister stated:

"Right now we have a limited range of options in treating aggressive forms of cancer. Those treatments, such as chemotherapy, can be effective but they can also be extremely toxic and difficult for patients. This compound offers the hope of a nontoxic therapy that could achieve the same results without any of the painful side effects."

Case History: Bradley Jones

"I'm a 39-year-old married family man with an 8-year-old boy and twin girls. I was diagnosed with bowel cancer in August 2008, with a tumor the size of an apple. During 2008 and November 2009 I took many conventional therapies including chemotherapy in tablet form combined with radiotherapy. As the weeks went by the side effects of the chemotherapy increased and it was hard to take the tablets knowing that they would make me feel worse. The radiotherapy burnt me so badly that my skin blackened and I could no longer walk. I recovered from these treatments and the tumor had reduced to the size of a pea. As it had reduced I could now have a procedure called Pappillion. This was a clinical trial and involved my tumor being zapped by a device that was inserted into my rectum. I endured three sessions and it was very, very painful. Three months later and my tumor was growing again. I now suffered another intrusive surgery called a THAMES; this involved them again going up my rectum but this time with a laser scalpel to cut the tumor away, after this operation I was informed that I should have a colostomy operation. After this painful operation I was subjected to more bouts of chemotherapy and after the third I felt as if I was dying. At the time, death would have been a welcome release. Over time I recovered and regular CT scans showed that I was cancer free, until one scan showed hotspots on my lungs; three on the left lung and two on the right. I was devastated! In February 2010 I had the bottom of my left lung removed. A biopsy found that it was bowel cancer that had spread to my lungs. I started to research other treatments for my condition and started to read about cannabis oil curing cancer.

I was very lucky to be put in touch with the authors of this book and I arranged to meet them. After asking me many questions I was given a syringe full of oil. Under guidance I took a small blob and swallowed it. The first effects could be felt within an hour, I felt the tightness and pain leave my chest and ribs and I could breathe more deeply and easily. I then began to feel a warm sensation and started to feel very stoned. I took the oil daily in small amounts four times a day and slowly increased the dose up to a gram a day. At my next meeting with my oncologist to discuss my latest scan results he informed me that the tumors on my right lung had reduced. I was lost for words. My new guardian angels again supplied me with another syringe of oil and I continued with the treatment. The oil also had a very positive effect on my anxiety and I did not feel at all anxious when I was taking it. I also managed to gain the weight I had lost from the chemotherapy. The oil gave me my appetite back and I gained enough weight to get back to a healthy and stable size.

Then came the news I'd been praying for: my wife and I attended an appointment with my oncologist and he commented on how well and healthy I looked. He seemed very pleased that I had put some weight on. After reading through my file he said, "The hotspots have reduced further on both sides at this moment in time. You are cancer free." Yet despite all this my oncologist isn't interested in the results I have achieved through use of cannabis oil. I feel totally let down by him and his attitude; he wasn't pleased or excited by my results and in fact he appeared lost and out of his depth. However, despite everything I am still cancer free and happy to report that cannabis oil has saved my life."

Clinical Endocannabinoid Deficiency (CECD)

Research has been carried out into many of the conditions that cannabis has been shown to successfully treat and according to a study by Ethan B. Russo, who is the Senior Medical Advisor to GW Pharmaceuticals, the company responsible for producing Sativex, the medical benefits of cannabis could be due to a deficiency in the brain's own endocannabinoid system, which closely mirrors the cannabinoids found in the cannabis plant.[36] The study examined the interesting concept that clinical endocannabinoid deficiency (CECD) could be the underlying cause of migraine, bromyalgia, irritable bowel syndrome, and other functional conditions alleviated by clinical cannabis.

Since the discovery of the human brain's own endogenous cannabinoid (endocannabinoid) system, we now have a better understanding of how cannabis may alleviate these conditions by boosting the body's own naturally produced cannabinoids and it may be that many of these conditions are in fact due to patients not producing enough cannabinoids themselves.

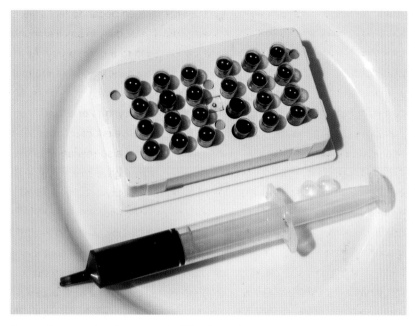

A capsule support makes accurate filling far easier.

Cystic Fibrosis

This condition is an inherited genetic disorder that is caused when two particular genes fail to function correctly. Symptoms include disruption of the endocrine glands that affect the pancreas, intestine, bronchial and sweat glands. Breathing and digestion are impaired by mucus. Medical cannabis use has been shown to reduce the severity of the condition and ease breathing (See Asthma).

Depression

There have been some controversial yet widely publicized studies linking depression to chronic use of cannabis. However, a peer-reviewed and well documented study that reviewed thousands of chronic, heavy cannabis users found normal rates of depression, once other factors such as alcohol use, gender and illness were accounted for.[37] It has been known for many years that depletion of the neurotransmitter serotonin in the brain leads to depression. Cannabis sativa varieties used in moderation have been shown to help combat clinical depression by increasing the production of serotonin.

When scientists looked at the overall death rates of research participants they discovered that those taking antidepressants had a 32% higher risk of death from other causes compared to non-users. In a survey, 72% of American doctors said they had prescribed antidepressants to children under 18, but only 16% of those said they felt comfortable doing so, and only 8% said they had adequate training to treat childhood depression. The United Nations has recently criticized the U.S. for overprescribing psychiatric drugs, as they consume 80% of the world's methylphenidate (generic of Ritalin).[38]

Antidepressants fail to help about half the people who take them, and a study in laboratory mice helps to explain why. Most antidepressants, including the commonly used Prozac and Zoloft, work by increasing the amount of serotonin, a message-carrying brain chemical made deep in the middle of the brain by cells known as raphe neurons. In January 2010 researchers at Columbia University Medical Center in New York reported that genetically engineered mice that had too much of one type of serotonin receptor in this region of the brain were less likely to respond to antidepressants. According to Columbia University's Rene Hen:

"These receptors dampen the activity of these (serotonin-producing) neurons. Too much of them dampen these neurons too much, it puts too much brake on the system."[39]

In October 2007 a new neurobiological study by Dr. Gabriella Gobbi of McGill University found that THC is an effective antidepressant at low doses.[40] However, at higher doses, the effect reverses itself and can actually worsen depression. This study offers the first evidence that cannabis can also increase serotonin, at least at lower doses. When laboratory rats were injected with the synthetic cannabinoid WIN55,212-2 and then tested with the Forced Swim test to measure "depression," the researchers observed an antidepressant effect of cannabinoids paralleled by an increased activity in the neurons that produce serotonin. However, increasing the cannabinoid dose beyond a set point completely undid the benefits.

Diabetes Mellitus

Diabetes refers to a group of metabolic diseases in which a person suffers from high blood sugar, either because the body does not produce enough insulin or because cells do not respond to the insulin that is produced. This produces symptoms including polyuria (frequent urination), polydipsia (increased thirst) and polyphagia (increased hunger). Medical cannabis use has been shown to help patients by stabilizing blood sugars, suppressing arterial inflammation common in diabetes sufferers, preventing inflammation of nerves and reducing the pain of neuropathy. It also acts as an antispasmodic agent, relieves muscle cramps and the pain of gastrointestinal disorders and acts as a vasodilator to help keep blood vessels open thereby causing lower blood pressure, which is vital for diabetics. Topical application of cannabis oil or cream has been shown to relieve neuropathic pain and tingling in hands and feet, and also reduce diabetic restless leg syndrome.

Dystonia

This is a severely painful neurological disorder causing involuntary muscle spasms and twisting of the limbs. A case study published in *The Journal of Pain and Symptom Management* reported improvement of the symptoms in a 42-year-old chronic pain patient, whose subjective pain score fell from nine out of 10 to zero following cannabis inhalation, and did not require any additional analgesic medication for the following 48 hours.[41] It is reported that no other treatment to date had resulted in such dramatic improvement in the patient's condition. Cannabidiol was given in doses, increasing from 100 to 600 milligrams per day, to five patients with idiopathic dystonia, along with previously administered treatments. Dose-related improvement ranging from 20% to 50% was noted in all patients.

Emphysema

Sufferers exhibit a gradual deterioration of the lungs caused by pollution and tobacco smoking. The lung air sacs become distended and rupture. Symptoms include breathlessness and blue lips. Cannabis aids in expansion of the bronchii and bronchioles allowing higher oxygenation in patients. This is not a cure but provides tremendous relief for patients (See Asthma).

Epilepsy

This is a medical disorder involving episodes of irregular electrical discharge within the brain, characterized by the periodic sudden loss or impairment of consciousness, often accompanied by convulsions. Cannabis is shown to reduce the frequency of attacks and researchers have discovered that three compounds found in medical cannabis can help to reduce and control seizures. CBD was tested on 15 epileptic patients, of whom 8 were given doses of 300mg. The remainder were assigned a placebo and treated for over four months, whilst continuing their past anticonvulsant drugs. Of the eight CBD-treated patients, four remained free of seizures, three showed partial improvements and one showed no response.

Fibromyalgia (FM or FMS)

People with fibromyalgia typically experience pain in their joints and muscles and may also suffer from frequent headaches and fatigue. This medical disorder is characterized by chronic widespread pain and allodynia, which is a heightened and painful response to skin contact or touch. Even light pressure is agonizing for many sufferers. This debilitating affliction causes aching muscles, sleep disorders and fatigue. Our bodies naturally make pain relievers called endorphins, but they also make other substances that can trigger pain relief in the endocannabinoid system. Fibromyalgia patients typically experience multiple areas of pain in the body and they often take multiple drugs for other symptoms, which can include difficulty sleeping, restless legs syndrome, depression, and anxiety. Cannabis uniquely has the ability to treat multiple symptoms. There is no known cure for fibromyalgia; it is notoriously difficult to treat and only 35–40% of people with the chronic pain condition get relief from the available medications. However, sufferers report a reduction in pain and improved sleep patterns from regular medical cannabis use. Lynda is a 48-year-old mother of three who lives in upstate New York, and was diagnosed with fibromyalgia in 2000. She is quoted on the website Health (.com) as saying, "I would use [cannabis] when the burning pains started down my spine or my right arm, and shortly after, I found I could continue with housework and actually get more done."

Glaucoma

This is caused by high pressure inside the eyeball that damages the optic disk. Typical treatments have serious side effects and have little effect on end-stage glaucoma. Cannabis lowers intraocular pressures dramatically, with none of the side effects, and is highly recommended as a treatment. When patients with ocular hypertension or glaucoma were tested with a dose of 19 milligrams of THC, seven out of 11 showed a 30% fall in intraocular pressure.

Glioma

This is the term for a tumor in the brain or spine. Malignant Glioma is very difficult to treat and the average survival time from diagnosis is only 40 to 50 weeks. THC has been shown to kill the Glioma cancer cells and is an effective treatment; many patients owe their lives to medical cannabis. A report published by the Department of Biochemistry and Molecular Biology based at the Complutense University in Madrid, with regard to cannabis and cancer treatment (particularly Glioma) states:

"Cannabinoids, the active components of Cannabis sativa L., act in the body by mimicking endogenous substances, the endocannabinoids that activate specific cell surface receptors. Cannabinoids exert various palliative effects in cancer patients. In addition, cannabinoids inhibit the growth of different types of tumor cells, including Glioma cells, in laboratory animals.[42] They do so by modulating key cell signaling pathways, mostly the endoplasmic reticulum stress response, thereby inducing antitumor actions such as the apoptotic death of tumor cells and the inhibition of tumor angiogenesis. Of interest, cannabinoids seem to be selective antitumor compounds, as they kill Glioma cells, but not their non-transformed astroglial counterparts."

Hepatitis C

Hepatitis C kills over 15,000 people in the U.S. every year, and whilst there is no vaccine currently available, there is new hope in nanoparticle technology.[43] More tests need to be carried out and the current treatment for hepatitis C still involves interferon medication. Its side effects can induce flu-like symptoms, fatigue, insomnia, loss of appetite, nausea, muscle or joint pain and depression. According to a report published in the October 2006 *European Journal of Gastroenterology and Hepatology,* a Northern California study involving 71 participants demonstrated that moderate cannabis use may relieve interferon's side effects, helping people with hepatitis C stick with the full treatment regimen.[44] Researchers state that cannabis's influence on hepatitis C is due to side-effect management, rather than an antiviral effect. Lead researcher Diana Sylvestre, MD, of the University of California at San Francisco emphasized that the benefit was primarily due to improved ability to stay on adequate doses of interferon and/or ribavirin.

Herpes

Herpes simplex is a viral disease from the herpesviridae family caused by both herpes simplex virus type 1 (HSV-1) and type 2 (HSV-2). Infection causes small, painful recurring blisters and inflammation, most commonly at the junction of skin and mucous membrane in the mouth, nose or genitals. THC has been shown to have a beneficial effect when used in the treatment of herpes. A topical application reduces the healing time of blisters and regular cannabis use reduces the frequency of attacks.

High Blood Pressure

High blood pressure can adversely affect the rate at which the heart works and is very destructive to the body. Poor sleeping patterns, diet, stress and overuse of alcohol can all contribute to an increase in blood pressure and cannabis use is helpful in relieving many of the causes of high blood pressure. Abnormally high blood pressure is known as hypertension and generally affects middle-aged men. However, most of us are going to suffer from cardiovascular disease at some point, as it is the number one cause of death in both men and women. Preliminary studies show that cannabinoids can lower blood pressure by dilating the blood vessels. This is despite cannabis use initially speeding up the heart rate in some users, thereby increasing blood pressure. However, for patients suffering from orthostatic hypertension or postural hypertension (a medical condition consisting of a sudden increase in blood pressure when a person stands up), cannabis use will actually cause blood pressure to lower.

HIV

Many people with HIV/AIDS use medical cannabis to combat wasting and other symptoms (See Anorexia Nervosa) and there are indications that cannabis use and a dietary supplement of hemp seeds has a positive influence on the body's immune system. Medical cannabis use for AIDS patients is proven to be beneficial, is extremely cost effective and offers an alternative for patients in third world countries who simply cannot afford expensive AIDS medicines. The supply of AIDS medication is big business. The pharmaceutical industry recently sued the South African government for breaking international patent laws. South Africa had tried to provide their desperately ill citizens with affordable copies of expensive AIDS medicines in a purely humanitarian act. The pharmaceutical companies indicated to the South Africans that they would be interested in helping them with the growing epidemic, providing it was shown to be financially beneficial.

Case History: Henry J. Sizluski, Jr.[45]

Henry has been living with HIV and herpes for over 24 years now. Previous to his cannabis use he was on pharmaceutical drugs that left him weak and his weight had dropped dramatically. He has relied on medical cannabis to help him deal with a variety of conditions, including the side effects of other medications. Cannabis has allowed him to reduce his dependency on pharmaceutical drugs and he now medicates with cannabis in tincture form, as well as smoking the buds from the plant. Henry has been able to regain the weight he had lost from wasting syndrome, and now has a correctly fitting prosthetic leg due to the increase in his body size, making it easier for him to walk again.

You can view Henry's full and informative video on the authors' website: www.cannabiscure.info/files/cannabis_treatment_3

Huntington's Disease

Disappointingly, a study by the University of Arizona found no improvement in Huntington's disease sufferers during a clinical trial that used only cannabidiol, not THC or the full profile of cannabinoids.[46]

However, research led by Dr. Javier Fernandez-Ruiz published in the *Journal of Neuroscience Research* studied the effects of both THC and CBD on Huntington's disease.[47] This study was not carried out on human patients but tested on rodents, and THC did show positive effects. In the human striatum (forebrain), CB1 receptors are the most common receptors for THC and Huntington's patients have been shown to have reduced levels of CB1 receptors in this area. Researchers administered high doses of THC to CB1-impaired rodents so as to over-activate their reduced CB1 receptors. It was shown that THC improved their motor function, slowed the disease symptom progression and improved the volume of their striatum.

Incontinence

Cannabinoids have been shown to reduce incontinence episodes without affecting voiding in patients with multiple sclerosis.[48] The study observed 630 patients who received either an oral administration of cannabis extract, THC or a placebo. Those receiving the active cannabis treatments showed significant effects over the placebo. The findings demonstrated a clinical effect of medical cannabis on incontinence episodes in patients with MS.

Inflammatory Bowel Disease

Medically, inflammatory bowel disease (IBD) refers to a group of inflammatory conditions of the colon and small intestine:

■ Ulcerative colitis is an inflammation of the colon that produces ulcer-ation of the inside wall. Its primary symptom is bloody, chronic diar-rhea, often containing pus and mucus, and associated with abdominal pain and weight and appetite loss. This is a chronic illness with no known cure.

■ Crohn's disease is an inflammation of the small and/or large intestine, with accompanying pain, cramping, tenderness, gas, fever, nausea and diarrhea. Though usually mild, in serious cases bleeding may occur and may sometimes be massive. This is also a chronic illness with no known cure.

■ Proctitis is an inflammation of the rectum and is characterized by bloody stools, a frequent urge to defecate but inability to do so and sometimes diarrhea.

Beneficial effects of cannabis treatment have been reported for appetite, pain, nausea, vomiting, fatigue, activity and depression. Patients also reported that cannabis use resulted in weight gain, fewer stools per day and less severe flare-ups. Patients not only report significant relief of their symptoms, but are also able to reduce the amount of prescribed immunosuppressive medications.

Insomnia

Cannabis has been shown to have a beneficial effect in helping sufferers or chronic insomnia, who report positive results from moderate consumption one hour before retiring. THC does not differ from conventional hypnotics in re-ducing rapid eye movement (REM) sleep. When THC was administered orally as a hydroalcoholic solution in doses of 10, 20 and 30 milligrams, subjects fell asleep faster after having mood alterations consistent with a high. Some degree of a hangover the following day follows larger doses. Ingestion can be very beneficial in treating insomnia and a dose of cannabis oil or an edible an hour before bed certainly benefits most sufferers.

Lack of Appetite (See Anorexia Nervosa)

One common side effect of taking cannabis is a powerful urge to eat, some-times known as the "munchies." Dr Kunos, scientific director of the National Institute on Alcohol Abuse and Alcoholism at the National Institutes of Health in the United States, carried out studies into the brain's own natural endo-cannabinoids to see if they had the same effect on appetite as cannabinoids in the cannabis plant.[49] Together with colleagues from Italy, Japan and the U.S., he found that, just like cannabis, natural endocannabinoids did indeed stimulate the appetite. This may go some way to explain why endocannabinoids are found in human breast milk and it is thought this has some function in stimulating babies to feed.

One of the most fascinating aspects of cannabis in relation to appetite is the effect of cannabis on body weight. Researchers have found that the cannabis can induce weight loss in those that are overweight and yet induce weight gain in people who are underweight. Currently no other drug can perform this dual function. Doctors can prescribe drugs for weight gain and weight loss but they cannot prescribe a drug that can do both.

Studies published in the *American Journal of Epidemiology* found that nationally in the U.S., rates of obesity were approximately one third lower in individuals who smoked cannabis at least three times a week.[50] The results were compared to people who have never used cannabis, and even after adjusting for other factors such as cigarette smoking, health, age and gender, the conclusion was that there is an inexplicable connection. Researchers analyzed data from over 52,000 participants in two large national surveys of the American population. The first survey found that 22% of those who did not smoke cannabis were obese, compared with just 14% of regular cannabis smokers. The second survey found that 25% of nonsmokers were obese, compared with 17% of regular cannabis users.

Leukemia

Leukemia is cancer of the blood cells. It starts in the bone marrow, the soft tissue inside most bones where blood cells are made. Studies have shown that THC kills leukemia cells. Cannabis oil is an effective treatment for this condition. Exposure of leukemia cells to cannabidiol has been shown to cause CB2-mediated reduction in cell viability and generation of leukemia apoptosis (programmed cell death).[51] Furthermore, cannabidiol treatment led to a significant decrease in tumors.

Methicillin-Resistant Staphylococcus Aureus (MRSA)

Cannabinoids are unaffected by the mechanism that superbugs like MRSA

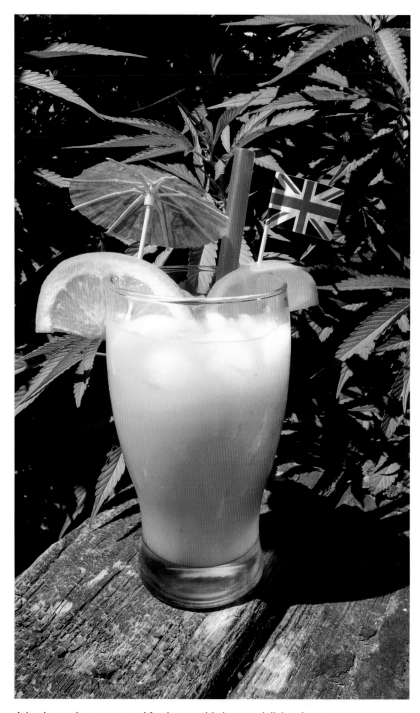

Juiced organic oranges and fresh cannabis leaves; delicious!

use to resist antibiotics. Scientists from Italy and the United Kingdom published research in *The Journal of Natural Products* reporting that cannabis-based creams could also be developed to treat persistent skin infections. [52]

Migraines

Many people confuse migraine headaches with cervicogenic headaches that arise from problems originating in the structures of the neck. Migraine headaches are usually unilateral (affecting one half of the head) and pulsating, lasting from 4 to 72 hours with symptoms of nausea, vomiting and sensitivity to light. It was once thought that migraines were initiated exclusively by problems with the blood vessels within the brain. However, the root causes of migraines are still unclear and there is new research that suggests they could be caused by CECD (see clinical endocannabinoid deficiency). Cannabis use is one of the most effective treatments for chronic, debilitating migraine attacks. Sufferers report that cannabis buds administered with a vaporizer give sustained relief within a very short period of time.

Multiple Sclerosis

MS is an autoimmune disease that affects the brain and spinal cord (central nervous system). In medical trials it was found that although THC does not halt the progress of multiple sclerosis, it does help to ease symptoms dramatically. Studies show that a dosage of 5 milligrams per day of THC produced relief from symptoms.[53] According to clinical trial data published in the *Journal of Neurology, Neurosurgery and Psychiatry*, "The oral administration of cannabis extracts significantly reduces muscle stiffness in patients with MS."

Muscle Spasms

An antispasmodic is a drug that suppresses muscle spasms seen in neurologic conditions such as cerebral palsy, multiple sclerosis, and spinal cord disease. Trials show that cannabis helps relieve peripheral muscular pain and cramping as effectively as pharmaceutical medications such as baclofen, tizanidine, and dantrolene, with no side effects. Clinical trials conducted by Jody Corey-Bloom, MD, PhD, of the University of California San Diego have shown smoking cannabis cuts spasticity and pain that is resistant to conventional therapy in multiple sclerosis (MS). Spasticity scores on the modified Ashworth scale dropped by an average 2.74 points more with smoked cannabis than with placebo.[54] A difference of 2 or more points is considered clinically meaningful on the 30-point Ashworth scale indicating mobility of elbows, hips, and knees. The trial included 30 patients with treatment-resistant spasticity randomized to double-blind use of a placebo cigarette or smoked cannabis, once daily for 3 days with crossover after an 11-day washout period. Pain scores, although relatively low to begin with at an average 12 or 13 points on the 100-point Visual Analogue Scale, fell by an additional 5.28 points with cannabis use. (Corey-Bloom J, et al - Smoked cannabis for spasticity in multiple sclerosis: a randomized, placebo-controlled trial). [55]

Nausea and Vomiting

Cannabinoids are extremely effective in treating nausea, vomiting and general sickness in many patients. It is particularly useful for cancer patients who choose to undergo chemotherapy and is recommended. THC is found to be superior to either Prochloperazine or Metoclopramide for pediatric cancer patients.[56]

Osteoporosis

Studies indicate that cannabis use may protect against osteoporosis, otherwise known as brittle bone disease. In normal bone growth, there is a balance between osteoblasts (the bone-forming cells) and osteoclasts (the bone-reabsorbing cells).[57] As we age, the osteoblasts slow down but osteoclasts continue to function normally and in some cases actually increase activity, which leads to the condition. Recently, the main components of the endocannabinoid system, namely the CB1 and CB2 receptors, along with the two main endocannabinoids, Anandamide and 2-AG, have been found in the human skeleton and they are reported to be involved in the regulation of bone metabolism.

CB1 receptor deficiency is believed to cause osteoporosis due to a marked increase in bone reabsorption, with an associated reduction in bone formation leading to increased fat cells in the bone marrow. During trials, this fat accumulation was prevented by cannabis use. Scientists now believe that the main physiologic involvement of specific CB2 receptors is to maintain a balance of bone remodeling, thus protecting the skeleton against age-related bone loss. Investigators at the Bone Laboratory of the Hebrew University in Jerusalem reported in the January 2006 issue of the *Proceedings of the National Academy of Sciences* that the administration of the synthetic cannabinoid agonist HU-308 slowed the development of osteoporosis, stimulated bone building and reduced bone loss.[58]

Pain Relief (Analgesia)

Prescription drug abuse is a pandemic problem in the United States today, with more than five million Americans now addicted to painkilling drugs such as OxyContin (oxycodone).[59] The analgesic or pain-relieving effects of cannabis are due in part to its chemical similarity to compounds produced naturally in the body, but without the potential for addiction. The endocannabinoids produced by our bodies are normally released by the brain under conditions of high stress or pain. Researchers at the University of California, San Diego School of Medicine, found that cannabis significantly reduces HIV-related neuropathic pain when added to a patient's already-prescribed pain-management regimen, and is an effective option for pain relief in those whose pain is not controlled with current medications.[60]

A further study was carried out by researchers from McGill University in Canada, funded by the Canadian Institutes of Health and published in the peer-reviewed *Canadian Medical Association Journal.* They reported that smoking cannabis from a pipe could significantly reduce chronic pain in patients with damaged nerves, adding that improvements in sleep and anxiety were also helpful to sufferers. In another unconnected study, THC administered intravenously to dental patients in doses of 44 nanograms per kilogram before undergoing tooth extraction was shown to produce a longer-lasting and positive analgesic effect compared to other analgesics, with no significant side effects noted.[61]

Cannabis is also known to make anesthetic far more "efficient," so if you are scheduled to undergo general anesthesia for whatever reason you are advised not to use any for at least 12 hours prior to the operation. If you are under the influence of cannabis, your anesthetist will panic as you will go too far under when they administer the drug. You can use as much cannabis as you require once the anesthetic has worn off.

Parkinson's Syndrome

Also known as Parkinson's disease, this is a degenerative disorder of the brain that leads to shaking (tremors) and difficulty with walking, movement and coordination. Cannabis is very effective at reducing, and in some instances completely stopping, the tremors and shaking (see Clinical Endocannabinoid Deficiency). The cannabinoids need to be taken at regular intervals to maintain the effect, and the condition is not cured by cannabis use, but it does provide relief from symptoms of sufferers.

In two patients with Parkinson's syndrome and coexisting dystonia who received doses of over 300 milligrams per day, it was reported that it exacerbated the hypokinesia and resting tremor, indicating there could be an aggravating action in such patients. [62]

Post-Traumatic Stress Disorder (PTSD)

Post-traumatic stress disorder is a severe anxiety disorder that can develop after exposure to any event that involves psychological trauma. Cannabis reduces the emotional impact of traumatic memories through synergistic mechanisms that make it easier for people with PTSD to sleep and feel less anxious, with reduced flashback memories. Whilst Israel allows medical cannabis use for any of its soldiers suffering from PTSD, an effort to persuade the U.S. administration to legalize cannabis for disabled war veterans who suffer from the condition was met with rejection from the White House. Gil Kerlikowske, Director of the Office of National Drug Control Policy, stated in June 201, that cannabis is not a benign drug and does not meet standards of safe or effective medicine.[63] This is incorrect.

One in five Iraq and Afghanistan veterans suffer from PTSD, and those who do seek treatment are prescribed expensive pharmaceutical drugs. Of these, nearly 20% will be given dangerous opioid-based narcotics like OxyContin and Vicodin instead of cannabis. According to a new study reported in The *Journal of the American Medical Association*, researchers found that whilst less than 7% of veterans without any mental health problems were prescribed addictive opiate painkillers, almost 18% with PTSD received a prescription for them.[64]

Opioid-based drugs are totally unsuitable for PTSD treatment and it is alarming that Vicodin is one of the top U.S. pharmaceutical products prescribed, when medical cannabis is far superior in terms of efficacy and cost. OxyContin is a $3 billion business and even more profitable than Vicodin for the pharmaceutical companies and their investors.[65] We can safely assume that the Office of National Drug Control Policy is fully aware of these statistics, and there is surely something morally wrong in denying combat veterans appropriate medication that not only works, but has been requested by the veterans themselves. PTSD has been recognized in combat veterans since Roman times, but it is only recently that the military has been forced to ad-

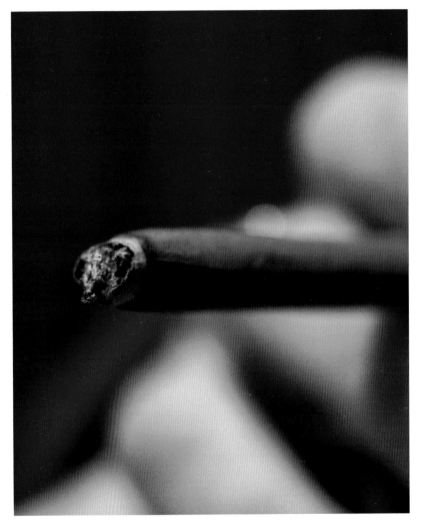

A "blunt." A cannabis joint rolled with a cigar wrapper.

dress the issue. It was found after the Falklands war in 1982 that returning British soldiers were badly affected by the brutal fighting and within ten years more veterans had committed suicide than died in the actual conflict.[66]

According to *HealthDay News* (March 2012), suicides among U.S. soldiers rose 80% from 2004 to 2008.[67] An Army study found that as many as 40% of these suicides may have been linked to combat experience in Iraq. Lead researcher Michelle Canham-Chervak, a senior epidemiologist, stated:

"Our study confirmed earlier studies by other military researchers that found increased risk of suicide among those who experience mental-health diagnoses associated with the stresses of war."

Michael Krawitz, Executive Director of Veterans for Medical Cannabis Access (VMCA) and a plaintiff in Americans for Safe Access v. Drug Enforcement Agency, admits that the Veterans association (VA) is trying to make progress. "The Army and Veterans Administration are trying their best to deal with these issues and have gotten pretty creative: employing meditation, yoga and even service dogs to assist [veterans] dealing with PTSD. But they haven't yet discovered cannabis."[68]

Premenstrual Syndrome

Premenstrual syndrome (PMS, also called PMT or premenstrual tension) is a collection of physical and emotional symptoms related to a woman's menstrual cycle. Studies indicate that moderate cannabis use can aid in the relief of painful stomach pains and cramps that are sometimes associated with this syndrome. It can also have a positive effect on a sufferer's mood and mental state.

Pregnancy

Current drug education literature still maintains that genetic damage is passed on by female cannabis users to their unborn children. This misinformation stems from unsubstantiated claims dating back to the late 1960s, when warnings that cannabis-caused birth defects were falsely predicted. Despite later studies disproving this, sponsored agencies continue to claim this as fact, citing studies carried out on rodents, where large doses of THC administered at specific times during pregnancy were shown to be detrimental. Because the effects of drugs on fetal development differ substantially across species, these findings are of no real relevance to humans, and studies with primates show no evidence of fetal harm from cannabis use. In one case, researchers exposed chimpanzees to high doses of THC for up to 152 days and found no resultant change in the sexual behavior, fertility or health of their offspring.

Research on human children examining the effects of prenatal exposure to cannabis have found no detrimental indications in cannabis-exposed babies in terms of health, temperament, personality, sleeping patterns, eating habits, psycho-motor ability, physical development or mental functioning. In fact other studies indicate that babies actually benefit from exposure to cannabinoids whilst in the womb. However, when researchers looked at black and Caucasian children separately, they found slightly lower scores on two subscales of the IQ test. In neither case did the frequency or quantity of the mothers' cannabis use affect the outcomes. This makes it extremely unlikely that they were actually caused by cannabis use. Nevertheless, this study is now cited as evidence that using cannabis during pregnancy impairs the intellectual capacity of children.

Melanie Dreher, RN, PhD, FAAN, coauthor of *Women and Cannabis: Medicine, Science, and Sociology,* is the Dean of the University of Iowa's College of Nursing and also holds the post of Associate Director for the University's Department of Nursing and Patient Services. She has honor degrees in nursing, anthropology and philosophy, and a PhD in anthropology from Columbia University. Alongside her achievements as a widely pub-

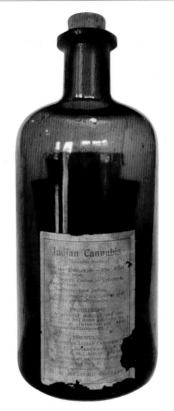

Cannabis was used as legal medicine until fairly recently.

lished researcher, writer and college administrator, Dreher is also a professor and lecturer at several institutions, including the University of the West Indies. She recently served as president of the 120,000-member Sigma Theta Tau International Nursing Honor Society and is an internationally well-respected academic.

Dreher has carried out an extensive study of pregnant women in Jamaica, which was later published in the *American Journal of Pediatrics* (1994) indicating that cannabis was being used in a cultural and medical context as a way to relieve morning sickness or nausea, prevent depression and fatigue, and to improve appetite.[69] Dreher acknowledges that such use is discouraged at Jamaican state prenatal clinics, but found that many women still consider cannabis to hold therapeutic benefits to both themselves and their unborn children. She studied a cross section of women who both used and abstained from cannabis during their pregnancy and then examined the babies one year after birth.

During the 30-day test period, it was expected that there would be a marked difference in the babies, specifically with regard to birth weight and neurological tests. Unexpectedly, it was discovered that children of the women who smoked cannabis regularly during pregnancy were more socially skilled, had better organization skills and improved sleeping patterns, were less prone to stress-related anxiety and made eye contact more readily. Those infants who had been most heavily exposed to cannabinoids indicated that:

- The quality of their alertness was higher.
- Motor and autonomic systems were more robust.
- They were inclined to be less irritable.
- They were less likely to demonstrate any imbalance of tone.
- They required less examiner facilitation to become organized.
- They displayed better self-regulation.
- They were more socially responsible and autonomically stable.

Dr. Dreher continues to argue against the restrictions placed on academics and scientists with regard to research concerning cannabinoid use during pregnancy, and objects strongly to the manner in which the public is deliberately misinformed. Furthermore, because women often face severe legal sanctions, including loss of custody, for admitting to cannabis use during pregnancy, most mothers refuse to divulge such information. Dreher recently wrote of how she had carried out an Internet search regarding pregnancy and cannabis. Typical

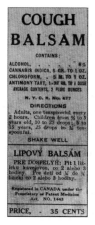

Cannabis medicine.

of the disinformation she found was an article entitled, "Exposure to marijuana in the womb may harm your fetuses [sic] brain." The article stated, "Over the past decade several studies have linked behavior problems and lower IQ scores in children to prenatal use of marijuana." This statement is both inaccurate and untrue.

Several major scientific studies have found that human breast milk naturally contains an abundance of the same cannabinoids found in cannabis, and one of its functions is to protect the cells against viruses, harmful bacteria, cancer and other malignancies. It has also been found that without these cannabinoids in breast milk, babies would not have the inclination to eat and promote growth. A study on the endocannabinoid receptor system published in the *European Journal of Pharmacology* (2004) states:

"Endocannabinoids have been detected in maternal milk and activation of CB1 (cannabinoid receptor type 1) receptors appears to be critical for milk sucking by apparently activating oral-motor musculature."[70]

A survey conducted by the directors of the Vancouver Island Compassion Society and the BC Compassion Club, published in the journal *Complementary Therapies in Clinical Practice*, reported that cannabis is therapeutic in the treatment of both morning sickness and hyperemesis gravidarum (a severe form of morning sickness, causing severe nausea and/or vomiting that prevents adequate intake of food and fluids).[71] Of the 84 women who responded to the anonymous questionnaire, almost half said that they had used cannabis intermittently during their pregnancy to treat symptoms of vomiting, nausea and appetite loss. Of these, 92% said that cannabis was "effective or extremely effective" in combating their symptoms and whilst most women chose to self-administer cannabis by smoking, 31% also reported benefit from consuming canna-edibles, and 8% reported using cannabis-based oils or tinctures. It is not recommended that any form of tobacco be used during pregnancy.

Premature Ejaculation

Premature ejaculation in men is conventionally perceived as "psychological." This seems less tenable when anecdotes support the claim that cannabis prolongs latency (time interval) and proof is apparent in the dose responsive delay in ejaculation in rats noted in experiments with HU 210, a powerful CB1 agonist. An agonist is a chemical that binds to some receptor of a cell and triggers a response by that cell.[72]

Australian research shows men who smoked cannabis daily were found to be four times more likely to have trouble reaching orgasm than those who did not, according to the La Trobe University study.[73] Professor Anthony Smith said whilst the habit often had a significant impact on a man's sex life, the effects were not always something the smokers would consider a sexual health problem. "The findings suggest that men are self-medicating with cannabis to delay orgasm," said Professor Smith from the Melbourne-based University's Australian Research Centre in Sex, Health and Society. The study took in more than 8600 people, aged 16 to 64, who were surveyed by telephone as part of the Australian Longitudinal Study of Health and Relationships.

Pruritus

This is chronic itching caused by a complex process involving different neurotransmitters, the hormonal system and blood vessels of the skin, psyche and other systems. Positive effects have been reported by a number of patients who have used cannabis to alleviate symptoms. Researchers at the Wroclaw University, Poland, investigated the effects of a cannabis-based ointment on 21 patients with pruritus due to end-stage failure of kidney function.[74] All patients applied the cream twice daily for a period of three weeks. Pruritus was completely eliminated in eight of the patients, with a noticeable improvement in the other test subjects.

Psoriasis

Psoriasis is an autoimmune disease that affects the skin. It occurs when the immune system mistakes the skin cells as a pathogen, and sends out faulty signals. Cannabis is used by many patients to treat psoriasis; the positive reaction is thought to be due to the anti-inflammatory properties of cannabinoids and their regulatory effects on the immune system. Regular topical applications of a cannabis-based cream or lotion can be beneficial and effective for many sufferers.

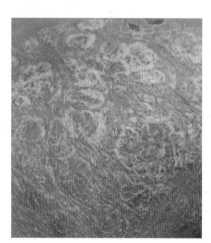 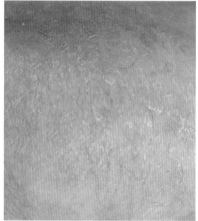

Left image shows the results of medically prescribed treatment with the chemotherapy drug Methotrexate. Side effects: Nausea, fever, diarrhea, abnormal liver function and increased risk of infection. Right image is the same arm treated with cannabis oil applied topically 3 times a day for 9 days. Side effects: Can now go swimming with her family for the first time.

Sickle-Cell Disease

Sufferers of sickle-cell anemia inherit a disease that is passed down through families, resulting in red blood cells forming an abnormal sickle or crescent shape within the body. Red blood cells carry oxygen and are normally shaped like a disc. Cannabis does not cure sickle-cell anemia, but is highly effective in managing pain. Cannabis also acts as a powerful anti-inflammatory without any side effects. The ocular (eyes and vision) effects of sickle-cell disease result from vascular occlusion, which may occur in the conjunctiva, iris, retina and choroid. Cannabis provides neuro-protective effects that may reduce the incidence of retinopathy and neuropathy.

Spinal Cord Injuries

Cannabinoids have been shown to be effective in reducing spasticity, and reports by individuals with these injuries have revealed a beneficial effect from cannabis use. The relaxing effect of cannabis on muscles in patients with spinal cord injury–related spasticity is due to an anti-spastic effect rather than a general relaxation response. According to data published in the *Journal of Neurotoxicity Research,* the administration of cannabidiol (CBD) improves mobility in rats with spinal cord injuries.[75] Investigators at the University of Sao Paulo in Brazil assessed the impact of CBD on motor function in rats with cryogenically (frozen) induced spinal cord injury.[76] The animals received injections of a placebo or CBD immediately before, three hours after and daily for six days after surgery. Researchers reported that cannabidiol-treated rats exhibited higher locomotor skills at the end of one week. Researchers reported, "Cannabidiol improved locomotor functional recovery and reduced injury extent, suggesting that it could be useful in the treatment of spinal cord lesions."[77]

Strokes

A stroke is extremely serious and can cause permanent neurological damage, complications and death. Risk factors for stroke include old age, high blood pressure, previous stroke or transient ischemic attack (TIA), diabetes, high cholesterol, cigarette-smoking and arterial fibrillation. Extracts from cannabis plants could have some efficacy in preventing brain damage after stroke, according to a team led by the British-born biologist Aidan Hampson at the U.S. National Institute for Mental Health in Maryland.[78] They discovered that THC and cannabidiol each act to prevent damage to brain tissue under laboratory

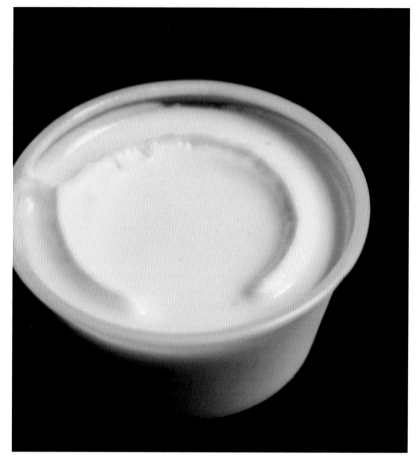

Cannabis oil-based cream for topical application.

conditions. Rats that were given cannabis decreased the size of their stroke by 50% and their brain injury was lessened by as much as 50%.

Tourette's Syndrome

This is a neurological disorder characterized by repetitive involuntary movements and vocalizations. In extreme cases, this condition causes the patient to move their limbs, shout, use inappropriate language and, in many cases, spit at people. It is very distressing for both sufferers and their families. There have been a number of studies investigating the therapeutic benefit of cannabinoids in treating tics associated with Tourette's. One of these studies (Muller-Vahl et al, 1998) found that when interviewed, 17 of 64 patients with tics admitted using cannabis, and 14 of these said that it reduced tics, pre-monitory urges and obsessive compulsive disorders (OCD).[79]

Another study reported a case report of a 25-year-old man with tics, ADHD, OCD and self-injurious behavior, who found that the use of tetrahydrocannabi-noid (THC) helped with many of these symptoms (Muller-Vahl et al, 1999).[80] A single dose of THC was shown to reduce his tic score on the YGTSS from 41 to 7, two hours after treatment. The patient also reported reduced premonitory urges and neuropsychological testing indicated improvements in signal de-tection and sustained attention. Medical cannabis has been shown to reduce the compulsion for patients to behave in socially unacceptable or inappropri-ate ways and control involuntary limb movement.

Ulcers and Warts

Ulcers can be cured internally by ingesting high-quality cannabis oil. External ulcers, warts and moles can be removed by topically applying cannabis oil and covering with a breathable plaster. The most effective coverings are the strips you cut to size yourself.

Acetone 99.9% purity

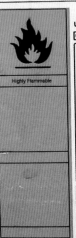

Highly Flammable

UN 1090

Batch No.

• Highly flammable. •
Keep out of the reach
of children. • Keep
container in a
well-ventilated place. •
Keep away from
sources of ignition - No
smoking. • Do not
breathe vapour. • Take
precautionary
measures against
static discharges.

Solvents Online Limited
Commerce Park, Frome,
Somerset. BA11 2FG
Tel: 01373 451170

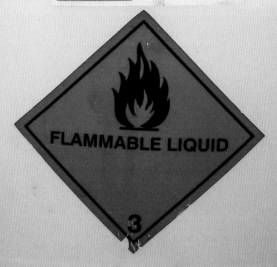

FLAMMABLE LIQUID

3

CHAPTER FIVE

Making Cannabis Oil

When properly made, cannabis oils are the ultimate extract for potency and purity. The oil is produced by adding dried cannabis plant material to a solvent, which is then evaporated off, leaving behind the extracted cannabinoid oil. There is an ongoing and wide-ranging debate as to which solvents and manufacturing methods produce the best oil; however, the method chosen will depend on your geographical location and the availability of suitable solvents for the extraction process. Regardless of the extraction method used, cannabis oil extracts are very versatile in their application.

Which Solvent?

We do not recommend using any particular solvent; your choice of solvent for an oil extraction will depend on local availability and your own personal preferences. The most common solvents used in the manufacture of cannabis oils are naphtha, acetone, butane, ethanol and isopropyl alcohol. Whichever solvent you choose, you must take care during the oil-making process as all these solvents are highly flammable.

All solvent evaporation MUST be done outdoors in a well-vented area, away from heat sources and naked flames!

Generally solvents fall into one of two categories: they are either polar or nonpolar. Polar solvents are soluble in water, and therefore they will also

Acetone is an organic solvent that evaporates rapidly.

extract water-soluble compounds from the plant as well as the cannabinoids. Nonpolar solvents are not soluble in water, and therefore they will extract less of the water-soluble compounds from the plant material. It is worth noting that acetone is an interesting solvent as it is classed as both polar and nonpolar. It is polar—that is part of the reason it mixes with water—but it is also soluble with non-polar substances like hydrocarbons.

One of the secrets to making high-grade oil extractions is the complete evaporation of the solvent: quality cannabis oils do not contain solvent. You must read the Health and Safety information supplied with the solvent and take great care when carrying out any extraction process.

All the solvents below will extract cannabinoids.

Acetone: Boiling Point 135°F (57°C)

Acetone is an organic solvent that evaporates rapidly, and for this reason it is considered by many to be one of the safest solvents to use for oil extractions. Acetone has a low toxicity if it is ingested or inhaled, and it is rated as a safe substance for food use as it is produced and disposed of naturally in the human body through normal metabolic processes. Acetone is both a polar and nonpolar solvent, which means that it will extract some additional compounds other than the cannabinoids from the cannabis material. It is available in various purities; if this is to be your solvent of choice then you are advised to seek out acetone of 99.9% purity.

Ethanol (Ethyl Alcohol or Grain Alcohol): Boiling Point 172°F (78°C)

Ethanol is the active ingredient in alcoholic drinks, and in its concentrated form it is an efficient solvent for making cannabis oils. However, due to the potential for abuse, many countries have restrictions on the strength and availability of strong alcohols and consequently they can be extremely difficult to obtain. For example, Everclear is a 190° proof (95% ABV) clear grain alcohol and the favored solvent for making F.E.C.O. (Full Extract Cannabis Oil). However it is only available in some American states.

Isopropyl (ISO) Boiling Point 180°F (82°C)

Isopropyl alcohol is generally more widely available and cheaper than ethanol. However, it is another polar solvent, so it will also readily dissolve the water-

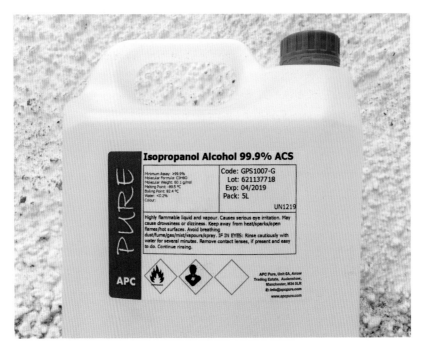

Isopropyl alcohol is another polar solvent.

soluble compounds from the cannabis plant material. Some oil makers feel that although polar solvents extract the cannabinoids sought, the extraction of the other substances is undesirable.

Even though we do not recommend any one particular solvent or process over another we recommend that you do not use Isopropanol (IPA) rubbing alcohol, as this contains additives to make it undrinkable. IPA can also contain detergents and dyes.

Naphtha: Boiling Point 86-194°F (30-90°C)

Naphtha is a colorless or reddish-brown, flammable hydrocarbon. Its characteristics are very similar to gasoline, and it is commonly used as lighter fluid or as a fuel for camping stoves. Generally speaking, less dense (lighter) naphthas will have a higher paraffin content. Naphtha may be carcinogenic, and frequently products sold as naphtha contain impurities which may also have harmful properties of their own.

Inhalation of naphtha vapor can cause symptoms of intoxication, and in severe cases it can be responsible for the depression of the central nervous

STEP-BY-STEP Crockpot Extraction

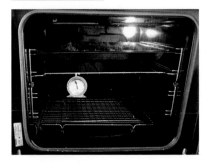

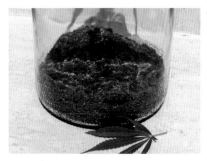

1. Completely dry the cannabis in an oven at 230°F.

2. Break up the dried bud, add your solvent, and shake or stir vigorously.

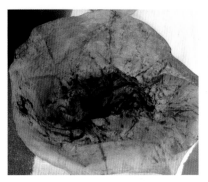

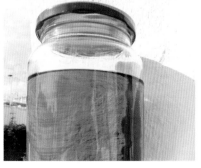

3. Filter the plant solvent mixture through a funnel lined with a coffee filter.

4. After being filtered it should be an amber-colored liquid.

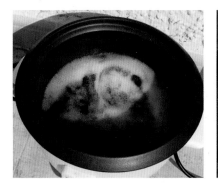

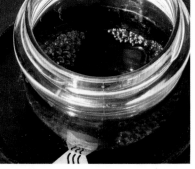

5. Pour the liquid into a crock pot or rice cooker with the lid removed and turn it on. The solvent will burn away. This is volatile and dangerous. Do it outdoors and away from open flames.

6. Once most of the solvent is evaporated pour the solution into a glass container and put it in a coffee warmer for the final evaporation process.

system. Symptoms of exposure can also include loss of appetite, muscle weakness, impairment of motor action, dizziness and drowsiness. Prolonged exposure to the skin can cause irritation; over exposure may also cause drying and cracking of the skin and associated dermatitis. People suffering from impaired respiratory function may be more susceptible to the effects of naphtha inhalation. As always, evaporate outdoors in a well-ventilated area.

Which Method?

When you have chosen your solvent, you will need to consider which method you are going to use to make your extraction.

The first step common to all methods is the decarboxylation of all the cannabis material to be used in the extraction. Decarboxylation is a chemical reaction that releases carbon dioxide (CO_2). When this occurs a chemical reaction takes place in which carboxylic acids loose a carbon atom from a carbon chain. This process converts the cannabinoid acids; For instance, THCA converts to THC, the psychoactive compound of cannabis. Gently heating activates all of the cannabinoids in this way and the better the quality of cannabis used, the better the resultant oil will be. Use top-grade cannabis buds for the best results and completely dry the cannabis in an oven at 230°F (110°C). Once the plant material has been removed and allowed to cool, take off all the stems and break the plant material into small pieces. This will allow the solvent to mix freely and ensure the efficient extraction of the cannabinoid oils. You should use enough solvent to completely cover and soak the cannabis plant material.

Crock Pot Extraction Method

This method uses a crock pot (slow cooker) to complete the solvent evaporation. You can also use a rice cooker to complete the process in the same way.

Place the bone-dry cannabis material into a container and cover with your solvent of choice. Shake or stir vigorously. The longer you agitate the mixture, the more cannabinoids you will extract. However, if you use a polar solvent like ethanol, then short exposures are preferred as polar solvents also extract water-soluble materials such as chlorophyll from the plant.

Filter the plant solvent mixture through a funnel lined with a coffee filter; if you are only making a small amount a cafetière is a convenient and quick way to remove the bulk of the plant material, but you still need to carry out the

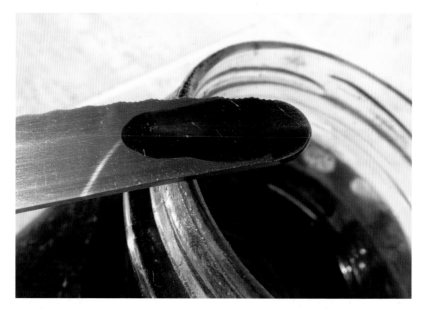

This is the finished product.

final filtration through a coffee filter which removes the empty trichomes and other fine contaminants. If you have filtered your solution correctly you will be left with an amber-looking liquid.

Pour the liquid into a crock pot or rice cooker and with the lid removed and turn it on. As the cooker heats up the solvent will start to boil away. Be careful, as boiling solvents are very volatile. This process must be performed outdoors in a well-ventilated area away from any naked flames.

Once the majority of the solvent has been evaporated, it should be poured into a glass container and placed onto a coffee warmer for the final evaporation process. This can take anywhere from 24 to 48 hours, and is complete when there is no more bubbling from the oil.

Allow the oil to cool slightly, and carefully draw up the oil into a clean syringe ready for storage or immediate use.

QWISO

This is an acronym for Quick Wash Isopropyl Oil, which literally means a "quick wash," typically taking under a minute. This method produces very high-quality oil with high cannabinoid content. Isopropyl alcohol is highly flammable so the final evaporation process must be carried out using a portable electric

STEP-BY-STEP Decarboxylated Cannabis Oil Production

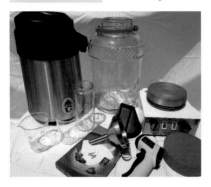

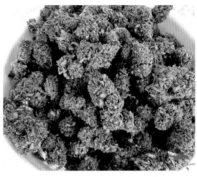

1. Equipment required: still or rice cooker; assorted glassware; funnels & filters; hotplate with variable temperature control; and laser thermometer.

2. For the best quality oil, use bud. You can use trim but your yield will be reduced.

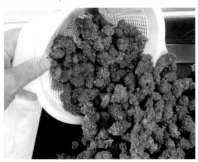

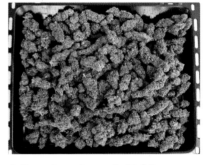

3. Dry plant material yields more oil.

4. Spread evenly on a baking tray.

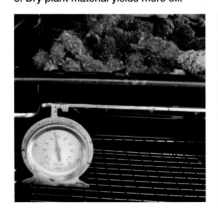

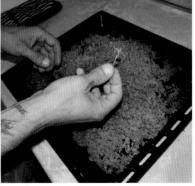

5. Dry in an oven. Max temperature 230°F (110°C).

6. When 'bone dry,' allow to cool before breaking up the bud, removing any large stems.

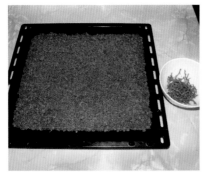

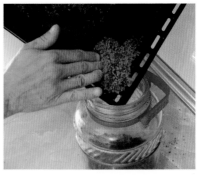

7. Ready for extraction.

8. Carefully place in a large glass jar.

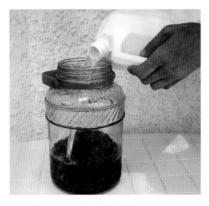

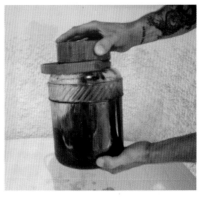

9. Add your solvent of choice.

10. Screw on the top and shake vigorously.

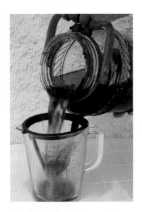

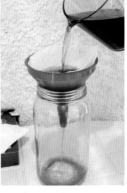

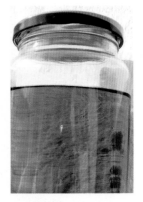

11. Pour through a sieve to remove the majority of the plant material.

12. Remove the finer particles by filtering through unbleached fine coffee filters.

13. After filtering you need to evaporate off the solvent.

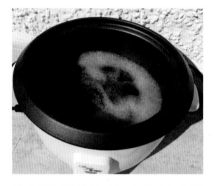

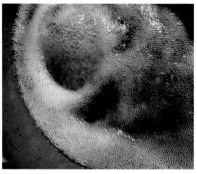

14. A rice cooker can be used to boil off your solvent. Always do this outdoors!

15. The boiling solvent will be very volatile and there is a risk of explosion. So, no naked flames!

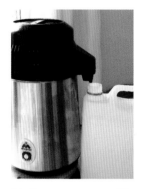

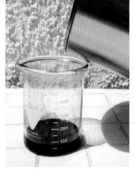

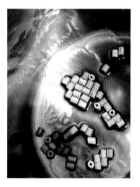

16. Or you can use a still to recover the majority of your solvent.

17. Switch off before all the solvent and (after leaving to cool) carefully pour into a suitable receptacle.

18. For this batch the authors used a still. The ceramic rings seen here aid the evaporation process.

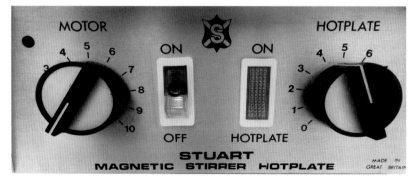

19. For the final stage, transfer the oil to a hotplate with variable temperature control. The authors use a magnetic hotplate stirrer. This useful device keeps your oil moving.

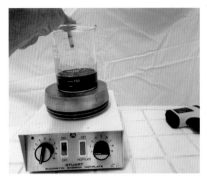

20. Dropping in a magnetic stirrer.

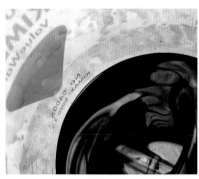

21. You can control the speed of the magnetic stirrer bar. Keeping your oil moving helps to avoid 'hotspots.'

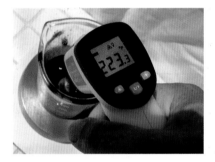

22. Once all your solvent has evaporated (after all bubbling has ceased), hold the temperature between 221°F (105°C) and 230°F (110°C) for 2 hours, after this your oil will be decarboxylated.

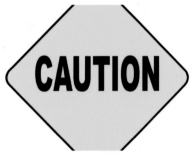

23. Avoid going above 248°F (120°C) or your oil will lose beneficial terpenoids.

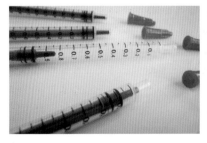

24. While the oil is still warm you can pull it into a syringe. These 1 milliliter syringes are great for administering small doses.

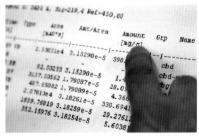

25. Having your oil(s) tested at a reputable laboratory and learning from the results is essential for the serious oil maker.

hot plate set up outside, or in a very well-ventilated area with no naked flames. For this technique, you will require a suitable quantity of isopropyl alcohol (99% purity), two large glass storage jars, a small flat Pyrex dish and a larger metal oven dish that the smaller Pyrex dish will fit into, along with a strainer and a coffee filter.

Break up your decarboxylated plant material and place it into a glass storage jar or similar container with a secure lid.

Next, pour on enough isopropyl alcohol to cover the plant material completely, and vigorously shake the jar for around 20 to 30 seconds.

ISO is a polar solvent, so only exposing the plant material for a short time limits the amount of chlorophyll and other water-soluble substances that may be extracted.

The mixture is then strained into a second container to separate the solvent from the plant material. Again, final filtration is via a coffee filter.

The liquid is then evaporated on a hot plate, or, if your hot plate gets too hot, place the Pyrex dish containing the solvent into a larger metal dish or bowl of hot water and place this on the hot plate.

Do not use a gas hob or any heat source with a naked flame as the fumes from the isopropyl alcohol can ignite.

You should be left with golden amber oil once the alcohol has been completely removed (when all bubbling has ceased).

Use a clean blade (a craft knife is ideal) to scrape and collect the oil.

Butane Honey Oil (BHO)

This is also referred to as honey oil and is made by using butane as a solvent, but this is a very dangerous process and must be carried out in a well-ventilated area, always outdoors! Butane fumes accumulating in a room can ignite from the slightest spark, even static electricity. There have been many instances of fires caused by people using butane as an extraction solvent and some fire departments in the U.S. have gone so far as to issue warnings against its use. There are many companies who sell ready-made butane gas extraction kits and they are readily available online. The best advice we can give is to not attempt this extraction process; if you decide to do so then wear protective clothing and always carry out the procedure outdoors away from any flame source.

Butane has a very low flash point (31.1°F or -0.1°C) and is most commonly used as a gas lighter fuel, but it is also extremely efficient at removing

STEP-BY-STEP BHO Production

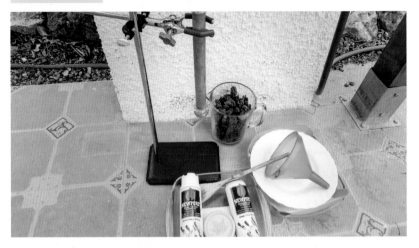

1. The equipment for making butane honey oil.

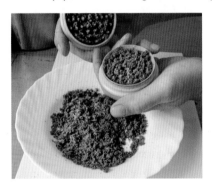

2. Grind up your bud.

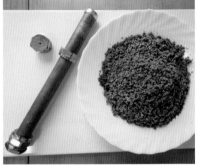

3. You can buy BHO extraction tubes or make your own out of a stainless steel pipe and fitting like the authors.

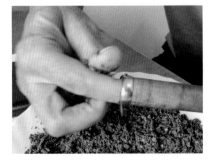

4. Load your extraction tube.

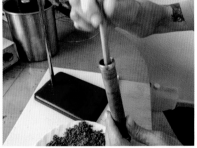

5. Pack the plant material, but not too tightly.

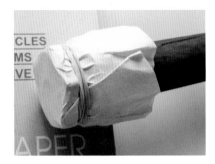

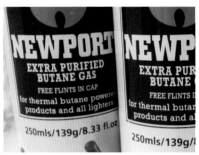

6. This homemade stainless steel tube has a 25 micron mesh filter but we also use a fine grade lab filter.

7. Use a high quality butane.

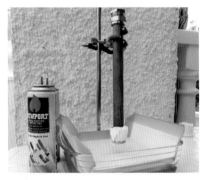

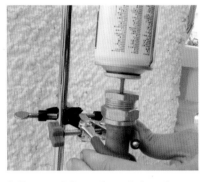

8. You can hold the tube in your hand but it will get very cold so use a stand.

9. Empty a full can through the tube. You may need more than one depending on the size of your extraction tube.

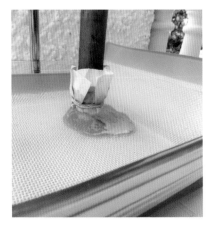

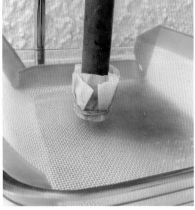

10. Collect the solvent in a shallow pyrex dish.

11. Looking good.

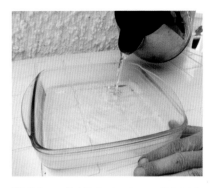

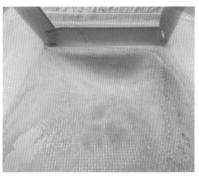

12. Take a slightly larger pyrex dish and fill with boiling water.

13. Place the dish with the butane on top.

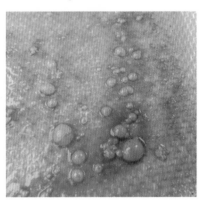

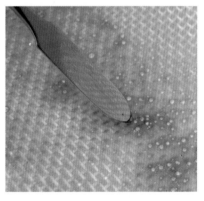

14. The heat from the hot water raises the temperature, thus aiding evaporation or 'purging.'

15. You can assist by 'pricking' and bursting the trapped butane.

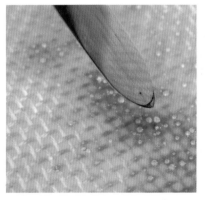

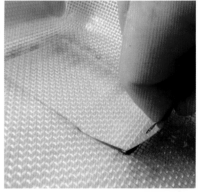

16. As time goes by, the bubbles will be fewer and smaller.

17. Use a clean 'blade' to collect your BHO.

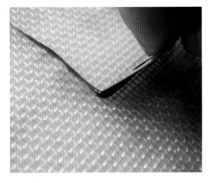

18. The oil mats are great.

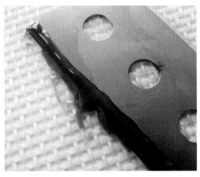

19. Still needs work.

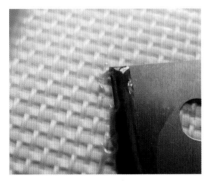

20. By working the oil 'manually' you can expel the remaining butane.

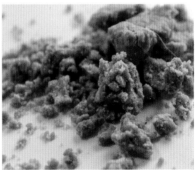

21. Good stuff!

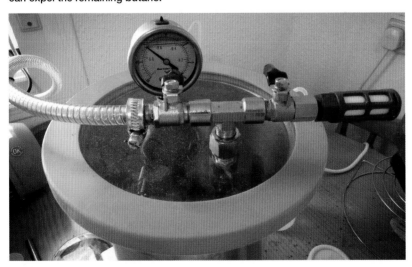

22. By using a vacuum chamber you can remove all the traces of butane to create 'shatter.'

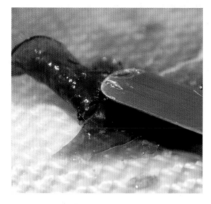

23. Getting there.

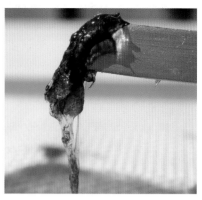

24. Made from Amnesia Haze bud.

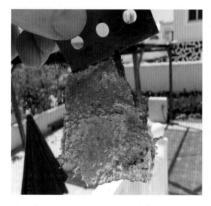

25. Would make a good sun filter.

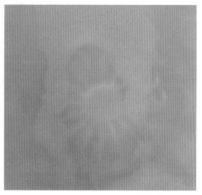

26. Butane evaporating.

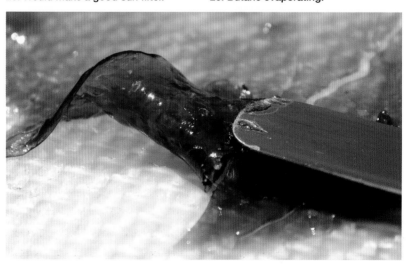

27. Final product.

cannabinoids from dried plant material. An important factor in BHO production is the purity of the butane: only use refined or purified butane gas.

The use of butane stove fuel should be avoided due to the addition of methyl mercaptan, which is added to aid the detection of leaks. This chemical also adds an unpleasant taste that is impossible to eliminate from the resultant honey oil.

Butane gases labeled as R-600 refrigerant or as refined or purified cigarette lighter fuel are generally free from contaminants, and these will produce the cleanest oils.

If you wish to carry out this process we do not recommend making the extraction tube yourself, as butane can affect many materials and it is also capable of dissolving some plastics. Glass is a safe material for BHO extractors and they can easily be purchased online and come with complete instructions.

The BHO process involves filling the extraction tube with very dry, finely chopped plant material through which butane is forced under pressure. As the liquid butane passes through the material in the tube, it dissolves the cannabinoid oils, and the resultant liquid is expelled from the tube to be collected in a Pyrex dish.

Owing to the low boiling point of butane, all that is needed to aid evaporation is to place the dish containing the liquid butane into a larger dish of hot water, but be careful to ensure that the hot water does not contaminate the butane in the Pyrex dish.

This extraction process produces very potent cannabis oil.

Making Concentrated Cannabinoid Oil Without Solvents

All of the solvents previously discussed have potential hazards associated with their use and/or the consumption of residual amounts contained within the oil extract.

It is possible to make concentrated cannabis oil without resorting to the use of solvents by infusing cannabis with an oil such as olive, sunflower or preferably cold pressed hemp seed oil. The drawback to this method is that the infused oil cannot be concentrated by evaporation; however, if you reduce the volume of plant material by making isolator (ice hash) first you can then produce a more concentrated oil.

In an article entitled, "Cannabis Oil: chemical evaluation of an upcoming cannabis-based medicine" - produced by Luigi L Romano and Arno Hazekamp from The Department of Pharmacy, University of Siena, Italy and The Plant Metabolomics group, Institute of Biology, Leiden University, The Netherlands, regarding the extraction of cannabinoids for medical use, they state:

"Of the solvents tested, this leaves olive oil as the most optimal choice for preparation of cannabis oils for self-medication. Olive oil is cheap, not flammable or toxic, and the oil needs to be heated up only to the boiling point of water (by placing a glass container with the product in a pan of boiling water) so no over-heating of the oil may occur. After cooling down and filtering the oil, e.g. by using a French coffee press, the product is immediately ready for

Concentrated Cannabinoid Oil Without Solvents

Preparation Time: 2 hours

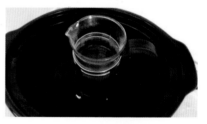

Equipment: Cafetière (French press)

Ingredients

- 100 grams of isolator (ice hash composing of unpressed trichomes, aka kiff, kief, kif)
- 200 milliliters Oil
- Pan of Water

Instructions

1. If you wish to retain the terpenes and prefer to consume the plants phyto-cannabinoids such as THC-A, et cetera, then there is no need for decarboxylation. If you wish to consume activated cannabinoids containing THC and CBD in its psychoactive form, then the Isolator must first be decarboxylated.

2. Half fill the pan with water and simmer.

3. Pour your oil into the cafetière and add in the Isolator hash.

4. Carefully place the cafetière into the pan of water

5. Leave for 2 hours, stirring occasionally.

6. Ensure that the pan does not boil dry and top up with water if required.

7. After 2 hours, allow to cool.

8. Remove the cafetière from the pan.

9. Slowly and carefully press the plunger.

10. Pour the concentrated infusion into a clean glass receptacle or jar.

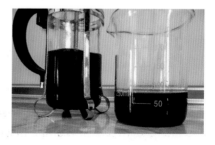

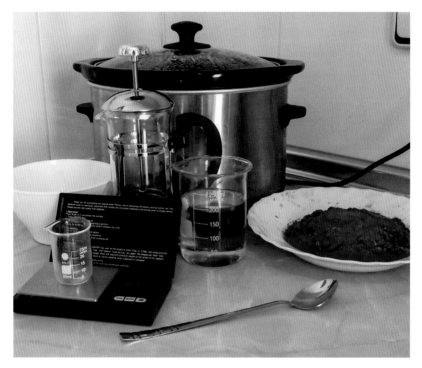

Some basic equipment required for extraction.

consumption. As a trade-off, however, olive oil extract cannot be concentrated by evaporation, which means patients will need to consume a larger volume of it in order to get the same therapeutic effects."

Dosage Calculator for Infused Oil

Depending on the quality and the strain, 1 pound (448 grams) of cannabis will produce around 2 ounces (55–60 grams) of concentrated cannabinoid oil if made with a solvent. This solventless oil extraction method using Isolator (ice hash) also requires a pound of cannabis flowers and this will yield in the region of 100 grams.

The 200 milliliters of infused oil used in this method contains the same amount of cannabinoids as 50 grams of concentrated oil made with a solvent.

How to Improve the Quality and Purity of Your Oils

In researching this book we have reviewed and studied hundreds of forensic and laboratory reports, with the most obvious conclusion being that the variance between the quality of the oil samples is the total amount of activated cannabinoids that are present.

To see if we could improve on some of the methodology, and therefore improve the quality of oil generally, we conducted a series of experiments in conjunction with the cannabis oil organization Bud Buddies. We submitted our oil samples to a reputable laboratory for analysis, and the results showed a distinct difference between the oils made with polar and nonpolar solvents, with the nonpolar solvents producing a better extraction. Acetone performed well despite having both properties. Nonpolar solvents do not readily dissolve water-soluble compounds, so plant matter can be exposed to these solvents for longer periods than polar ones without extracting any unwanted contaminants.

One of the easiest ways to improve on the quality of your oils is to filter correctly. Poor filtration means contamination and that reduces the quality of the end product. Poorly filtered oils also burn easily, whereas correctly filtered oil will not burn on a coffee-warming hot plate. The addition of unwanted contaminants results in heat being absorbed, which raises the temperature and can cause your oil to burn. Filtration through the coffee filter takes a long time, but this step is essential in all cannabis oil preparation.

As polar solvents like ISO and ethanol also extract water-soluble compounds, you can reduce the amounts extracted by freezing the cannabis and the solvent. To be really effective, you also need to freeze the receptacle used in the extraction process. By freezing, the cannabinoid oils are extracted but the water-soluble elements remain in the frozen plant material. The solvent is then strained and filtered before the extraction process.

You can also increase the purity of oil made with polar solvents by reducing the amount of plant material used in the extraction. The cannabinoids are all contained within the trichome, so by removing the trichomes you drastically reduce the amount of plant material and therefore the amount of solvent required is also dramatically reduced.

Ice-Water Separation aka Isolator (Bubble Hash)

This is an extraction technique for separating the trichomes from the cannabis plant material. This process requires ice, water and agitation and filtration bags with variously sized screens. Cannabinoids are insoluble in water, but if you place cannabis plant material into cold water, the trichomes will become brittle. If they are then agitated, they will be dislodged from the plant into the cold

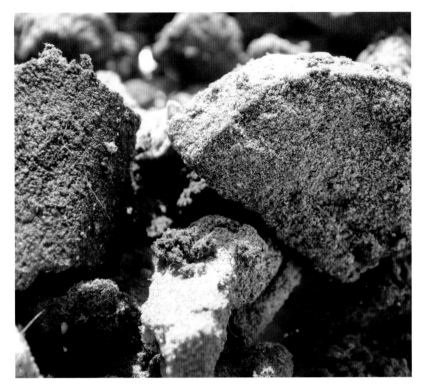

Bubble hash.

water. Ideally, the temperature should be one or two degrees above freezing and this is achieved by adding plenty of ice to the water during the process. The cold water is then strained through the various bags that have very fine mesh screens in their base. The first bag in the system is a mesh of around 220 microns (a micron is a millionth of a meter), which removes the majority of the plant material. The trichomes are collected by the remaining bags, which have smaller meshes. Some of the finest screens are as small as 25 microns, and these finer screen grades produce very potent bubble hash. This hash can then be further processed to make a high-quality, medical-grade oil.

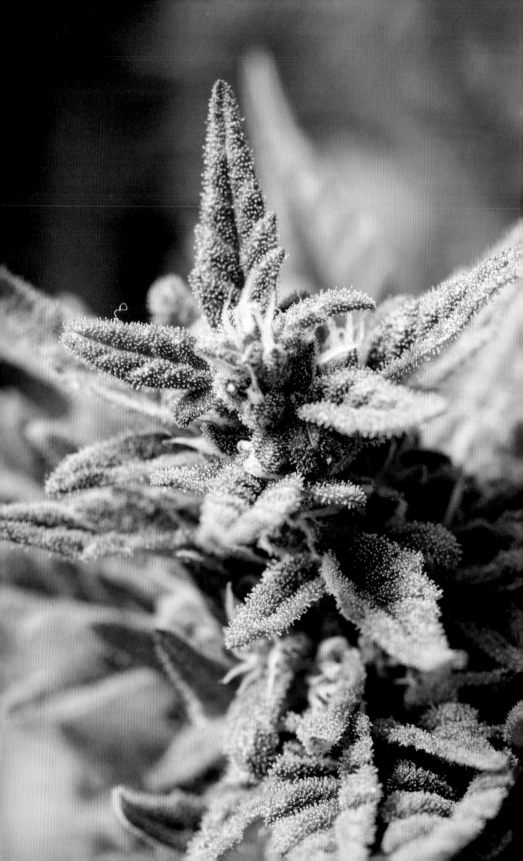

CHAPTER SIX

Hemp Nutrition and Health

The importance of good nutrition in maintaining optimum health cannot be overemphasized, considering the modern Western diet. As Dr. Alejandro Junger stated, "The problem is we are not eating food anymore, we are eating food-like products."[1] We are the descendants of hunter-gatherers, and our ancestors primarily ate vegetables, fruit, nuts, seeds, roots, fish and meat. This diet was high in healthy fats and protein, but low in grain and sugar-derived carbohydrates. The average person's diet today is not what we have evolved to live on and we now suffer more chronic and debilitating diseases than ever before. Particularly within Western society today, a large percentage of people are overfed and undernourished with large amounts of trans fat, refined sugar, cereal, bread, potatoes or pasteurized milk products comprising their diet. Eating a diet that is high in trans fat can raise the level of cholesterol in the blood increasing the risk of cancer and heart disease. Although traditional medical advice, based on a decades-old, misconstrued study by Nathan Pritikin, led many of us to believe that saturated fat was the enemy of good health and a major cause of heart disease, it is now thought that saturated fat is essential for good health-especially of the brain, cells, liver and for effective absorption of vitamins and minerals as well as protection against disease. Modern studies show that in fact trans fats (unsaturated fats with trans-isomer fatty acids), excessive consumption of carbs and sugars and a

....

It's not just the buds of the cannabis plant that are good for your health.

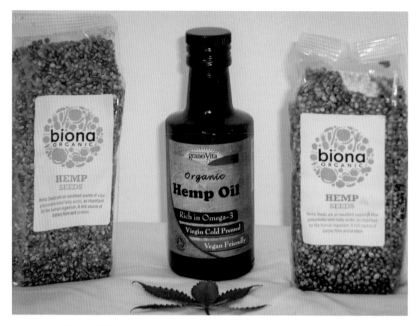

Commercially available hemp seed and oil.

diet low in fat can be incredibly dangerous. The proliferation of processed food into our modern diets has caused many of the medical issues mentioned above, and the obsession with "low-fat" alternatives to fatty products means that sugars and carbs sneak into our diets under the guise of being healthy. A diverse diet based in unprocessed, whole foods with good quality fats and proteins, healthy grains and pseudocereals, lots of fruit and vegetables and limited amounts of sugar is your best bet for a healthy body–and hemp can be an important part of such a diet.

It was not until the 20th century that obesity became a global health issue, and the World Health Organization recognized it as a worldwide epidemic.[2] In 2008, the organization estimated that 1.5 billion adults were overweight, and of these, over 200 million men and nearly 300 million women were obese.[3] Obesity is defined as an abnormal or excessive fat accumulation that may impair health; a body mass index (BMI) greater than or equal to 25 is classified as overweight, and a BMI greater than or equal to 30 is labeled obesity. Furthermore, in 2010, more than 40 million children under five were categorized as overweight. The American Institute for Cancer Research's second expert report, Food, Nutrition, Physical Activity, and the Prevention of Cancer: a Global

Perspective, confirms the relationship between excess body fat and increased cancer risk.[4] According to the scientific literature, there is convincing evidence that body fat increases risk for cancers of the esophagus, pancreas, colon and rectum, endometrium, kidney, and breast cancer (in postmenopausal women).

The Healing Seed

The seed of cannabis sativa L. has been an important food source and medicine for thousands of years. Eaten raw, the cannabis seed was certainly used by prehistoric humans, yet, as a direct consequence of prohibition, the true potential of this super food has not been exploited to any great extent within Western culture. The ancient Chinese medical text *Pen-Tsao Kang-Mu* states, "The Ancients used this medicine to remain fertile, strong and vigorous."[5] The compiler of this epic Chinese Materia Medica, Li Shih Chen (1518-1593), writes that in ancient times, varieties of ma zi (the hemp seed plant) were readily distinguishable from drug crops. One variety originated on Mao Luo Island in the Eastern Sea, and its seeds were reported to be as large as those from the lotus plant.

Hemp seeds can be successfully used as part of a healthy, calorie-controlled diet, and have been found to leave individuals feeling more energetic, fuller and far less likely to crave starches, carbohydrates or sugary snacks.

Hemp can be grown in poor soil and produces an abundant crop within a short growing season. If used to its full potential, it could be of real benefit in areas suffering from food shortages. The plant is easily grown without pesticides or herbicides, and besides its highly nutritious seed, it yields a strong fiber that can be used for weaving cloth and utilized as a building material for the construction of shelters. Hemp can be fertilized with organic waste, and if fertilizer is properly applied, the crop may be grown for decades on the same soil with no corresponding drop in yield. If it can't be grown in a region that requires food aid (due to drought, civil unrest or warfare), it can be imported cheaply as it is light to ship and easy to prepare. Yet as a food resource it is suppressed, undervalued and largely ignored in the West, although hemp seed has long been valued as a nutritional food source throughout Asia, India, Russia and Eastern Europe. In Russia, hemp seed is used as a substitute for dietary fats such as butter and hydrogenated margarine. In China, street vendors still sell roasted hemp seeds that are purchased as a popular snack, and houmayou, a soup containing hemp seed oil, is traditionally eaten twice a day in some rural areas. Hemp seed has always been part of the Japanese diet and can be found in Asian restaurants and grocery stores as shichimi, used for seasoning, and asanomi, which are basically tofu burgers with a hemp seed coating. Cannabis is still used in rural Cambodia and Laos to flavor soups, but generally it is the stalks and leaves that are used in much the same way as Westerners would use herbs.

The meat of the shelled hemp seed resembles that of other cultivated grains, including wheat and rye, and does not contain any psychoactive compounds. Hemp seeds can be eaten raw, ground into a meal, sprouted, made into nondairy milk products, prepared as tea, brewed into beer or used in cooking. They are obtainable as a legal food product and becoming increasingly available in North America and Europe. Products now readily obtainable include cereal bars, pasta, muesli, bread, waffles, hemp tofu, a variety of spreads and hemp nut butters, along with bottled hemp seed oil.

Technically classified as a nut, cannabis seed contains rich translucent oil, high in amino and fatty acids, which are 90% unsaturated. However, if you wish to benefit from the full profile of amino acids, it is better to consume hemp seeds uncooked as some amino acids are destroyed by heating. The seeds typically contain around 33% protein, second only to soy (35%), but are more easily digestible and their primarily globular proteins are one of the most complete forms of protein available from plants. Hemp seed's overall protein content of over 30 grams per 100 grams of seed is better than that found in nuts, other seeds, dairy products, fish, meat or poultry. Hemp protein also has high arginine content, typically 123 milligrams per gram of protein, and histidine at 27 milligrams per gram of protein. Arginine is classified as a semi-essential or conditionally essential amino acid, whereas histidine is an essential amino acid for humans. It was initially thought that it was only essential for infants, but longer-term studies established that it is also essential for adults. Hemp seed is also high in the sulfur-containing amino acids methionine at 23 milligrams per gram of protein and cysteine at 16 milligrams per gram of protein, which the body needs for proper enzyme formation. Hemp seeds also contain a high antioxidant content in the form of alpha, beta, gamma, delta-tocopherol and alpha-tocotrienol.

Essential nutrients are not produced by the body and must be obtained from a dietary source. Nonessential nutrients are those nutrients that can be made by the body, but these are also absorbed from consumed food. The

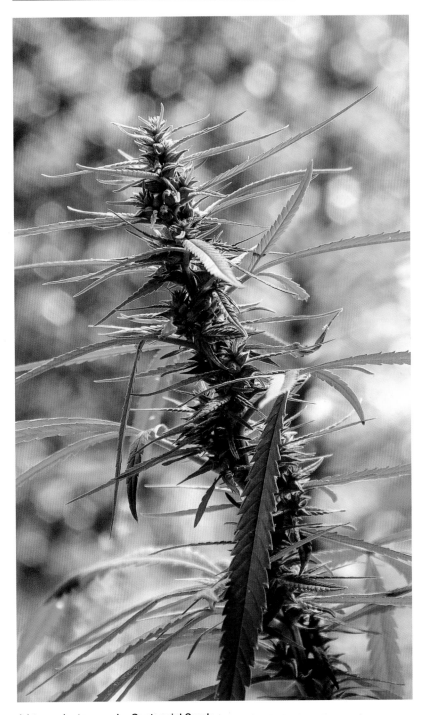

A hemp plant grown by Centennial Seeds.

majority of animals ultimately derive their essential nutrients from plants. For humans these include essential fatty acids, essential amino acids, vitamins, and certain dietary minerals.

No one food source has them all, but hemp seed comes close, and its amino acid profile is almost complete when compared to more common sources of protein such as meat, milk, eggs and soy. It has an omega-3 content even higher than walnuts, which contain 6.3%.

Once harvested, the seeds not destined for sale as hemp nut are cleaned and cold pressed in a dark and oxygen-free environment to preserve the product. This produces high-quality polyunsaturated oil and crushed seed hulls known as "seed cake," which can be ground into flour that is 41% protein but gluten-free, and which has been approved by the U.S. Celiac Society as a safe ingredient for anyone suffering from gluten allergy. No known allergies exist to hemp foods and the fat content of shelled hemp seed is relatively low compared to other nuts and seeds. Hemp food products have low cholesterol content and contain high concentrations of natural phytosterols that have a well-documented cholesterol lowering effect.

Hemp Nut (Hulled Hemp Seed)

Another process, called "de-hulling," removes the seed coat, leaving the hemp nut. There is no significant difference in the medicinal or nutritional content of hulled hemp seeds, they are simply more convenient to use and can be purchased cheaply online. They can be consumed alone, or used instead of other grains, seeds and nuts in recipes. Only 6.6% of the total calories in shelled hemp seed come from saturated fat compared to 14% of saturated fat calories common in the modern diet.

The hemp nut consists mainly of oil, typically around 44%, 33% protein and dietary fiber and 12% other carbohydrates (predominantly from residues of the hull). In addition, the nut contains vitamins, particularly the vitamin E complex, phytosterols and trace minerals. Overall, hemp's advantage over other seeds is its fatty acid profile and its protein, which contains all of the essential amino acids in nutritionally significant amounts and in a desirable ratio.

Most oil seeds contain linoleic acid (LA), an essential fatty acid (EFA) from the "omega-6" family, yet they offer little alpha-linolenic acid (ALA), the other EFA from the "omega- 3" family. Humans should ingest these EFAs in an omega-6/omega-3 ratio of about 4:1.

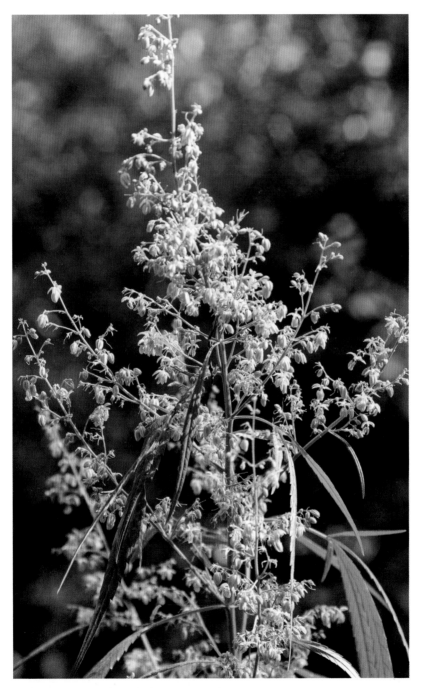

Another hemp plant grown by Centennial Seeds. Industrial hemp producers can use male plants like this for many different purposes.

Since seed oil and animal fat, both low in omega-3, account for most of our fat intake, Western diets typically have omega-6/omega-3 ratios of 10:1 or more, which is far too rich in omega-6 and correspondingly too deficient in omega-3. This imbalance is a cofactor in a wide range of common illnesses, including cardiovascular diseases, arthritis, diabetes, skin and mood disorders.

Hemp Seed in Traditional Medicines

Hemp seed has been used in Traditional Chinese Medicine (TCM) for more than 2000 years and is known as *Huo Ma Ren*. It is still employed today as a recuperating energizer and for tonification *(bu fa)*, which is a treatment designed to address poor functioning of the body's vital organs. In Chinese culture, *qi (chi)* forms an essential part of any living being and is the central underlying principle in TCM; *qi* is frequently referred to as life force, life energy or energy flow, and practitioners regard any deficiency of this energy as the main cause of disease in the body. This deficiency is also referred to as asthenia syndrome in Western medicine, which is represented medically by a number of different conditions, including: lack of muscle strength, sickness, dizziness or fatigue. This can result from inherited factors present at birth or acquired factors such as poor diet, emotional disturbance, chronic and major illness, childbirth, environmental influences or aging. Hemp seed is prescribed for the treatment of many ailments, but is said by the Chinese to particularly help moisten and nourish the intestines, spleen and stomach. It is prescribed to treat constipation, aid recuperation after fever, disease or childbirth and the seed is believed to nourish the body's Yin (the dark force opposing Yang in Chinese philosophy), remove heat from the body (high temperatures and fever) and promote healing of sores (taken orally or applied topically as hemp seed oil).

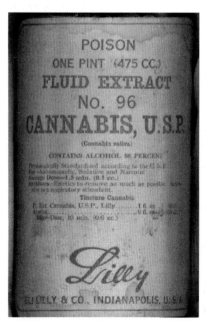

Cannabis was readily available as medicine, prior to prohibition.

Ayurveda (Ayurvedic) is a system of medicine that originated in India several thousand years ago. The term Ayurveda combines two Sanskrit words: ayur, which means life, and veda, which means science or knowledge. Ayurveda literally translated means the science of life. Hemp seed is known as Vijaya Siddhi. Vijaya means "victorious" and cannabis is said to be victorious over many illnesses and diseases. Hemp seed and hemp seed oil are prescribed in Ayurvedic medicine as a demulcent laxative (meaning an agent that forms a soothing protective film when administered onto a mucous membrane), an anti-inflammatory, and a nervous system restorative, as well as a cardiac tonic to reduce low-density lipoprotein (LDL) cholesterol levels and fatty deposits. It is similarly prescribed for the treatment of ulcers and inflamed mucous membranes. As oil, it is recommended to reduce inflammation in eczema, psoriasis and acne.

The basis of Ayurvedic medicine are the three doshas: Vata, Pitta and Kapha. The doshas are general body types and basically refer to small, medium and large, but dosha also specifies the patterns of how our bodies use energy. Vata spends energy, Pitta manages it and Kapha stores it. Hemp seed's Ayurvedic actions are referred to as Snigdha (demulcent), Rasayana (rejuvenating), Anuloma (redirecting the flow of Vata downwards) and Vibandha hara (alleviating constipation). When the doshas are balanced the body is said to be in homeostasis (a state of zero change), and this is considered to be the perfect state of health.

Further Benefits of Hemp Seed

A study published in the *Journal of International Medical Research* reports that hemp seeds have successfully been used to treat atherosclerosis, eczema and ADHD. They are also a useful bulk-forming laxative that can improve the frequency and consistency of stools. Furthermore, according to the University of Michigan, hemp seed extract contains an unidentified compound that is thought to help boost learning and memory function, as well as enhance the immune system.[6] Researchers there discovered that hemp seeds stimulate a brain chemical called calcineurin, which plays a key role in healthy brain synapse activity. The *Journal of Pharmacology, Biology and Behavior* published the results of a study that showed that calcineurin increased both brain and immune function in mice. A follow-up study showed that calcineurin could repair learning and memory skills that had been previously affected by chemical drug addiction.[7]

The high amounts of omega-6 and omega-3 fatty acids, as well as the phytosterol content, found in shelled hemp nut are known to have a beneficial

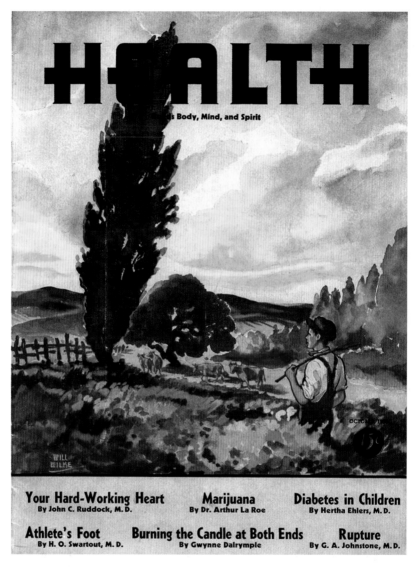

H✝ALTH

Body, Mind, and Spirit

Your Hard-Working Heart
By John C. Ruddock, M.D.

Marijuana
By Dr. Arthur La Roe

Diabetes in Children
By Hertha Ehlers, M.D.

Athlete's Foot
By H. O. Swartout, M.D.

Burning the Candle at Both Ends
By Gwynne Dalrymple

Rupture
By G. A. Johnstone, M.D.

The health benefits of cannabis have always been recognized.

effect on cardiovascular health, by reducing blood cholesterol levels, reducing arterial thrombosis and decreasing the thickening of artery walls with fat deposits that cause atherosclerosis. Furthermore, phytosterols have been shown to reduce total serum cholesterol by an average of 10% and low-density lipoprotein (LDL) cholesterol by an average of 13%. Phytosterols may offer protection against colon, breast and prostate cancers.

A diet containing the correct balance of omega-6 to omega-3 fatty acids may also help delay or reduce neurodegenerative disorders such as Alzheimer's and Parkinson's syndrome. Additionally, gamma-linolenic acid (GLA) contained in hemp seed has been found to be effective in treating rheumatoid arthritis and active synovitis, and may also be helpful for osteoporosis sufferers. There is further evidence to suggest a beneficial role for hemp seeds in combating irritating skin disorders.

As the oil in hemp seed is known to inhibit platelets (tiny cells that help with blood-clotting) anyone taking anticoagulant drugs should be aware that there is a theoretical possibility that bleeding could occur. This is only speculative; if there is an issue it is caused by the toxic pharmaceutical drugs, not hemp seed. Overdose or drug interactions with the oral anticoagulant warfarin (Coumadin) can lead to lethal toxicity, as can exposure to super-warfarin (also known as long-acting anticoagulants). Warfarin is the primary toxic agent used in rat poison; rodents that ingest it crawl away and bleed to death from all orifices. If you are taking toxic anticoagulants you are advised to consult your physician before starting any hemp seed treatment.

Recommended Dosage

The typical minimum dosage of raw hemp seed in treatments is between 10 and 30 grams per day. They can be eaten raw, sprinkled on cereal and toast or mashed and powdered before being added to food or drink mixes. This amount is confirmed by the University of Michigan, who recommend that the dosage of shelled hemp seed is 15 grams or one heaped tablespoon twice daily.[8] There is no potential for overdose unless you are taking warfarin, and this dosage can be supplemented with additional hemp seed in your meals, snacks and salads. You can take up to 60 grams a day, which is four heaped tablespoons, and this is the recommended maximum. If you do overindulge on hemp seed products, be aware that it can have a laxative effect. If this is unwanted, simply eat less. The proportion of linoleic and alpha-linolenic acid in one tablespoon (15 milligrams) per day of hemp seed oil can also readily provide all of the body's daily requirements of Essential Fatty Acids (EFAs).

Cannabinoids are produced within the glands of the cannabis plant itself, so the seeds do not contain any significant amounts of psychoactive compounds. Cannabis seeds from drug crops are also cannabinoid free, although occasionally tiny particles of resin can stick to the seed casing resulting in minor traces. However, this does not apply to commercial hemp seed. It is physically impossible to experience a high from using hemp seed or hemp seed oil, even when it has been heated. Studies have been conducted to examine if hemp products could adversely affect consumers required to undergo mandatory drug testing in the workplace. Over a trial period volunteers were given a selection of foods containing hemp nut. The results indicated that none of the volunteers had cannabinoid levels consistent with recreational cannabis use.

Hemp Seed Smoothies

One of the easiest ways of consuming hulled hemp seeds is in smoothies. Just mix a tablespoon of organic hulled hemp seed with fruit and juice of your choice in a blender. You can optionally add yogurt to produce a thicker consistency. This makes a good protein shake with a complete dose of amino acids and EFAs. Protein is one of the fundamental building blocks of muscle and is particularly recommended for those who are exercising on a regular basis. Athletes, bodybuilders and sportsmen especially can benefit from hemp-based drinks that are a nutritious alternative to dairy or soy-based protein supplements.

Hemp Balls (Nai Lao Yi Qi)

This recipe appears in the ancient Chinese Pen-T'sao Kang-Mu, and as well as helping to restore qi energy, it is also recommended to stave off hunger for long periods. The cooking process will destroy amino acids, but as it is one of the first recorded medicinal treatments using hemp seed it is worth mentioning.

Ingredients

- 2 quarts hulled hemp seed
- 1 quart soy beans

1. Boil together until soft, drain and then heat gently in a pan, stirring frequently until they become dry.

2. Remove them from the heat, allow them to cool and then grind into a powder with a mortar and pestle or coffee bean grinder.

3. Combine with a small quantity of honey to act as a binder; add small amounts and stir the ingredients together in a bowl until the mixture reaches the required consistency.

4. It should adhere together but not be overly sticky. Hand roll the substance into small balls. These are eaten twice daily. If you wish to experiment with this recipe, we recommend that the minimum size you make each ball is one ounce in weight (28 grams).

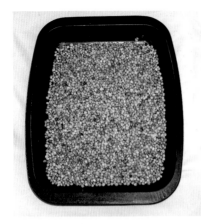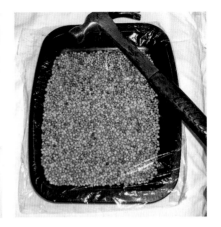

Hemp seed placed into a baking tray either for toasting to make a tasty snack or to crush the seeds to remove the hull. To dehull simply cover with clear film and gently crush the seeds with a hammer.

Hemp Nut Salad

Salads are a great way of eating your 2 tablespoons of raw hemp seeds a day. Simply sprinkle 1 tablespoon of hulled hemp seed per portion of tossed salad. It is recommended that organic hemp oil be used in the dressing. Try 1 part hemp oil, 1 part white vinegar and the juice of a freshly squeezed lemon. Increase or reduce the quantities to taste, and season with ground black pepper.

Toasted Hemp Seeds

Heating damages the amino acids contained within the seeds, but this snack is a far healthier alternative to potato chips or pretzels. Toast your hulled hemp seeds in a pan until light brown, and add salt and pepper to taste.

Hemp Seed Weight-Loss Plan

If you consume more calories than you are using, your body will store fat. If you are overweight you can lose one to two pounds of body fat per week following this simple diet. Hemp seed is used to provide a filling and healthy alternative protein. If you are obese or have any condition that may be affected by dieting please consult your physician beforehand, but this is a sensible eating plan and will ensure the fat stays off. A calorie-controlled diet is the most effective way to lose weight and maintain a healthy Body Mass Index (BMI); you will live longer, suffer fewer illnesses and have more energy. You

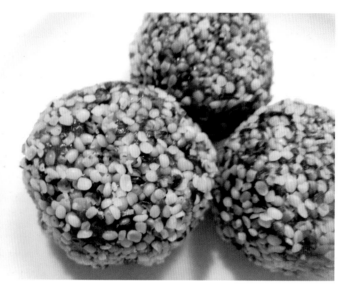

Delicious and healthy hemp seed balls.

Hemp Balls: A Contemporary Recipe

These are a modern twist on Hemp Balls (Nai Lao Yio Qi) and can be made with cannabis-infused olive oil, but our recipe uses commercially available hemp oil. The balls are designed to be used by patients who suffer from digestive problems and can be used as a complete meal replacement.

Preparation Time: 5 minutes.

Ingredients:
- 4 cups hulled hemp seed
- 4 cups of oats
- 3 cups desiccated or grated raw coconut
- 1 cup raw sunflower seeds
- 1 cup hemp oil
- 400 grams honey

- 4 cups hemp flour to dust the finished balls. This can be purchased from any good health food store. Hemp seeds do not mill into flour readily; they become butter because of the high oil content. In order to get flour, you need to remove the oils.

1. Mix the ingredients thoroughly, lastly adding the honey as a binder. It is preferable to first put the hemp and sunflower seeds through a coffee bean grinder if you have one, but this is optional.

2. Divide the mixture into 24 servings and hand-shape into round balls. These will be slightly sticky and can then be coated with the hemp flour.

Makes 24 servings.

Hemp Milk

Organic hemp milk is a legal, healthy alternative to dairy milk. You can purchase the ready-made product in good stores, but it is cheap and easy to make yourself. Fresh-shelled hemp seed milk has a white to slightly green or gray appearance and a pleasant taste. You can experiment with flavors by adding almonds, vanilla or figs, which all complement the taste of hemp nut.

Preparation Time: 2 minutes.

Ingredients:

■ 1 cup shelled hemp seeds (hemp nuts)

■ 5-6 cups cold water (previously boiled and allowed to cool)

1. Combine the water and hemp nut in a blender. You can create the desired thickness by using more or less water.

2. Blend on a high-speed setting for 2 to 3 minutes, or until creamy and smooth.

3. To strain (if required): pour the blended mixture through a cheesecloth and squeeze into a bowl. You should be left with a thin coating of pulp on the inside of the cloth, which you can rinse off.

4. To sweeten (if required): add fruit, maple syrup or honey. Blend until smooth. Optionally you can then strain the milk again through a cheesecloth.

Hemp milk will keep for three days if refrigerated in a sealed container.

Makes: 6-7 cups.

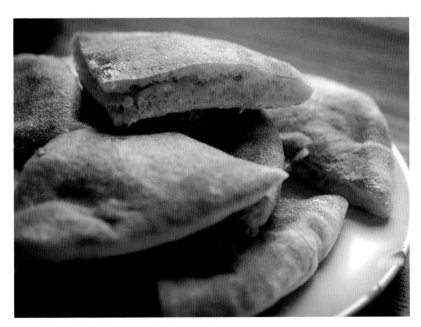

Tasty cannabis edibles; bread with cannabutter is a great treat!

don't require any fad diet books or expensive weight-loss supplements. Most of these fad diets shed pounds very quickly, but nearly all of them do not have a lasting effect. The pounds that seem to drop off so miraculously are mostly bodily fluids lost through dehydration. In fact, some studies have shown that as many as 90% of all dieters regain the weight within a year of losing it and many put on even more weight.

Simply count your calories by using either an inexpensive food calorie guidebook or Googling a free online guide. Plan your three meals a day with breakfast being the most important; eat less in the evening if you can. Write down the calorie content of each meal and add up the total.

An average man requires around 2,500 calories a day to maintain his weight. For an average woman the figure is around 2,000 calories a day. These values can vary depending on age and levels of physical activity. The ideal calorie intake to lose weight is at least 500 calories below maintenance level, and never more than 1000 calories below. There are approximately 3,500 calories in a pound of stored body fat. So, if you create a 3,500 calorie shortage over the course of a week, you will lose one pound of body fat.

Cut out red meat, sugar, alcohol, processed foods, white bread, pasta and dairy products completely. Replace potatoes and white rice carbohydrates with raw hulled hemp seeds, legumes, whole grains and other fresh vegetables. Whole grains such as brown or wild rice, oats, barley and rye, or foods made from them, contain all the essential parts and naturally occurring nutrients of the entire grain seed and are a good source of fiber. Quinoa, amaranth and buckwheat are classified as "pseudo-grains" but are normally listed alongside true

Hemp Nut Coleslaw

Delicious, healthy and nutritious coleslaw can also be made with raw ingredients.

Preparation Time: 5 minutes

Ingredients:

- 1 cup of shredded red cabbage
- 1 finely chopped clove of garlic
- 1 finely chopped chili (optional)
- 1 chopped red onion
- 1 chopped scallion, chopped fresh parsley or cilantro
- ¼ cup of hulled hemp seeds
- 2 tablespoons of hemp oil
- salt and pepper to taste.

1. Combine the ingredients in a salad bowl and toss well.

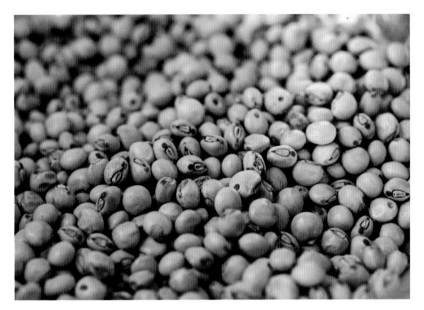

Hemp seed.

cereal grains because their nutritional profile, preparation, and use are so similar.

Legumes are also high in fiber and are classified as plants with seed pods that split into two halves. Edible seeds from plants in the legume family include beans, peas, lentils, soybeans, and peanuts and these should all be included in your diet plan.

Be cautious of eating too much fruit as they contain sugars in the form of fructose. It is possible to realize a healthy diet without fruit, but fruit does make it easier to achieve certain vitamin levels. Fruits high in sugar include: tangerines, cherries, grapes, mangos, figs and bananas. Low sugar fruits include: lemon, lime, rhubarb, raspberries, blackberries and cranberries.

Replace your fish and poultry protein as often as you like with raw hemp seeds. If you are a vegetarian, simply include hemp seeds with your fresh vegetable dishes. There are only 340 kcal per 60 grams of hulled hemp seeds, which equals your four heaped tablespoons a day, and eating a good breakfast that includes hemp seeds should leave you free of significant hunger until mid afternoon.

Drink plenty of water. Most people are unaware of how much water they should be drinking daily and many of us are in a constant state of dehydration without even realizing it. The process of burning calories requires an adequate supply of water in order to function efficiently and dehydration slows down the fat-burning process. Studies have produced varying recommendations over the years, but realistically your water needs depend on many factors, including your health, how active you are and where you live. The Institute of Medicine has determined that an adequate intake for men is roughly 3 quarts (about 13 cups) of total beverages a day and for women, 2.3 quarts (about 9 cups) a day.

It is important that you add an exercise regime to boost your weight loss. Walk more, take the stairs not the elevator, ride a bicycle, jog or swim if you can, join a gym or exercise at home. If you are obese, ill or unfit please consult your physician before exercising. Losing weight utilizing hulled hemp seeds really is as simple as this.

Hemp Seed Oil

This healthy and nutritious oil is increasingly becoming available in grocery stores and health food shops. It has all the benefits of hulled hemp seeds and is also one of the best known sources of the Essential Fatty Acids omega-3 and omega-6. Hemp oil is also a rich source of vitamins A and E, which are powerful antioxidants. Unlike flaxseed oil, hemp oil can be used continuously without developing a deficiency or other imbalance of EFAs and the ratio of the two EFAs is 3.38, closely approximating the 4.0 average ratio recommended by the World Health Organization. In addition, the biological metabolites of the two EFAs, gamma-linolenic acid (18:3 omega-6; "GLA") and stearidonic acid (18:4 omega-3; "SDA"), are also present in hemp seed oil. Hemp oil also has effective anti-inflammatory properties. Anywhere you use regular cooking or dressing oil you can use hemp oil. Its nutty flavor and light texture are perfect for salad dressings, sauces or drizzling over vegetables. It is the preferred oil for many internationally acclaimed chefs, and is both full of natural enzymes and cholesterol-free.

Juicing Raw Cannabis

Raw cannabis contains THCA (A refers to acid) and CBDA, which must be heated to produce THC and CBD. This is the reason for decarboxylating or simply smoking the dried flowers. Test results show that heating converts 300 milligrams of non-psychoactive THC acid into 5 milligrams of psychoactive THC, and whilst the 5 milligrams retains its medicinal value it is a small percentage of the original THCA. THC acid isn't psychoactive in its raw state but still has ther-

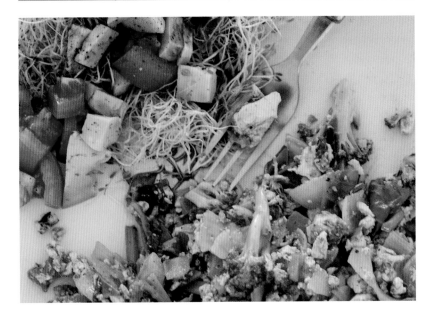

Hemp oil makes a superb salad dressing.

apeutic value and patients can gain much higher concentrations of the non-psychoactive cannabinoids without experiencing the associated high. However, THCA converts naturally into THC, and therefore it is important that only fresh leaves are used if the aim is not to ingest the psychoactive THC compounds.

While there are close to 70 cannabinoids known to have therapeutic effects, CBD is quickly becoming the second most important (after THC). Most of the varieties today contain large amounts of THCA which, when heated, provides THC. CBDA-dominant strains are being developed, but the main problem faced by medical users, who either purchase their cannabis on the black market or grow from seed, is the lack of consistency in strains. Identically named strains from different breeders can have differing cannabinoid content. David Suzuki, the academic, science broadcaster and environmental activist asserts that cannabis grown for recreational purposes is found to contain increasingly high levels of THC and little CBD.

According to Dr. William Courtney, an MD from California, cannabis leaves contain the highest CBDA levels and are best harvested when the plant is between 70 to 85 days old. After 90 days they rapidly produce more THCA. CBDA has been proven to treat many medical conditions and acts as an anti-inflammatory, antibiotic, antidepressant, antipsychotic, antioxidant, a sedative

STEP-BY-STEP Cannabis Juicing

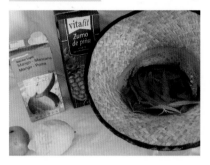

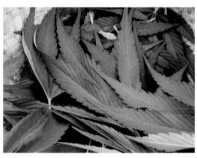

1. Preparing the ingredients for juicing fresh, raw cannabis fan leaves. You can also just add fruit juice.

2. Freshly picked fan leaves from an organic plant. Choose only leaves with a healthy color from a vigorous plant.

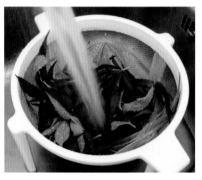

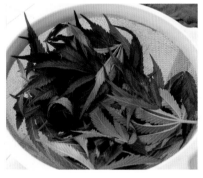

3. The collected fan leaves are placed into a colander and thoroughly washed under running cold water.

4. The freshly washed leaves are removed from the running water and shaken to remove any excess liquid.

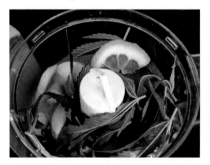

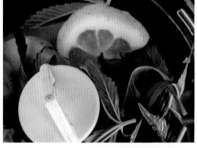

5. The leaves are placed into the blender along with any fruit or vegetables you wish to add. You can experiment with different flavors.

6. For this juice we have added a few slices of fresh, organic lemon, apple and a small amount of chopped fresh ginger.

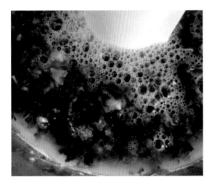

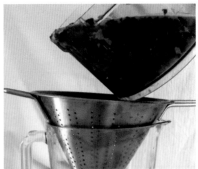

7. The ingredients are thoroughly blended together in the juicer for 1 to 2 minutes.

8. Place a colander into a good size jug and strain the freshly blended ingredients. Squeeze the remaining pulp.

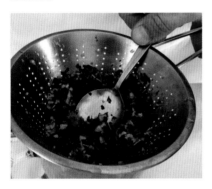

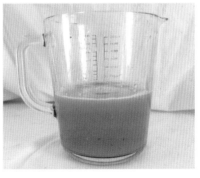

9. Here we are using the back of a spoon to squeeze the remaining pulp but you can also simply squeeze the pulp by hand.

10. The juice can be consumed as it is or used as a base for delicious and healthy fruit juice cocktails.

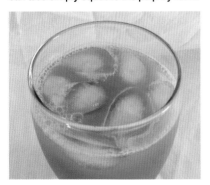

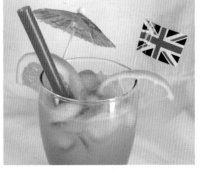

11. Ice can be added to the fresh juice to make a healthy and refreshing summer drink.

12. Fresh orange juice has been added, but you can use any combination and carrot juice works well.

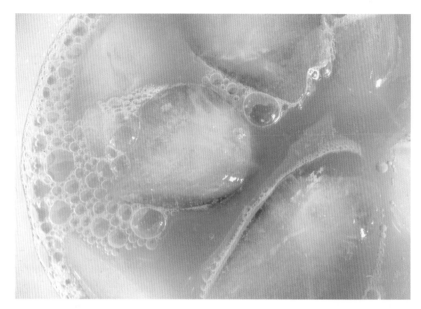

Cannabis infused juice.

and is believed to have beneficial immune-modulatory properties. It has also been shown to relieve convulsions, inflammation, anxiety and nausea, and inhibit cancer cell growth. However, patients can also obtain this benefit from CBD, and this is delivered far more effectively through vaporizing or the use of medicinal cannabis oils produced by extraction.

Dr. Courtney is one of the main proponents of the raw cannabis juicing treatment and has presented anecdotal evidence of the benefits, claiming that at least one patient has benefited tremendously from its use. This patient is his wife Kristen and her story is undoubtedly remarkable.

Kristen Courtney was suffering from joint inflammation and an array of autoimmune conditions, including interstitial cystitis and lupus, that caused her organs and other tissues to swell.[9] She was prescribed over 40 different anti-inflammatory, antibiotic and painkilling medications in an unsuccessful attempt to combat the symptoms and had developed steroid toxicity. She was told by her doctors that she might possibly make it to her thirtieth birthday. In desperation, Kristen moved to California, where she could legally grow her own medicine, and began juicing cannabis leaves on a daily basis. Kristen's condition improved significantly, and today her pain has been completely eliminated and she has stopped using any other painkillers. Kristen's story is available to view on YouTube.

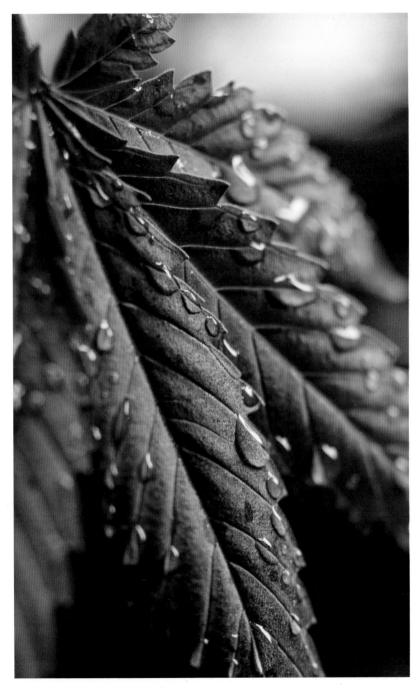

Do not use any leaves that appear discolored or over fertilized. The plant should not be in flower. Vigorous growth is indicated by these healthy looking cannabis leaves.

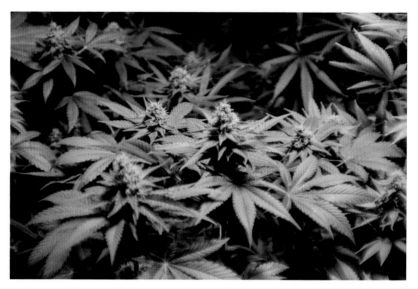

Lush green foliage on flowering plants.

However, Michael Backes of the Abatin Wellness Center in California, a well-respected medical cannabis dispensary backed by state-of-the-art analytical testing, stated in response to Dr. Courtney's claims:

"Dr. William Courtney has been researching juicing cannabis for several years. The young woman in the video, Kristen, is his wife. Courtney makes some very plausible points, but his claims really do need to be subjected to randomized, controlled clinical trials. Courtney's claim that raw cannabis is not psychoactive is true, but only for pristine, fresh cannabis.[10] Disturb the gland heads on a living cannabis plant of a strain that contains THC and the process of converting its non-psychoactive THCA to psychoactive THC begins, albeit slowly."

Professor Manuel Guzman, from the Complutense University in Madrid, is involved in the study of how the active components of cannabis (the cannabinoids) act in the body, with special emphasis on the molecular mechanisms of that action, and on understanding how cannabinoids control cell generation and death.[11] We have some involvement with the professor and specifically asked him the following question with regard to ingesting raw cannabis:

"Phytocannabinoids produced by the plant do not bond with cannabinoid receptors, so when they are ingested fresh from an immature plant, what exactly are they doing in the body, if anything?"

His response does give some validation to the juicing theory:

"Yes, most (but not all) of the cannabinoids in the fresh plant are carboxylated and bind to CB1 and CB2 cannabinoid receptors with low (but some) affinity. Then it is not an all-or-none issue. In addition, carboxylated THC may bind to additional as yet unknown molecular targets beyond cannabinoid receptors in the body. In short, the fresh plant is clearly less psychoactive than the treated/cured plant, but we still have to learn much more on the pharmacology of carboxylated cannabinoids."

In response to the same question, Dr. Paul Hornby, a very well-respected authority in biological and biochemical science stated:

"In answer to your question, nobody knows, since it's never been thoroughly studied, but judging from the biochemistry of the cannabinoid molecules, even if not activated (decarboxylated) and may not bind the receptor, they still are antioxidants, anti-microbial and have some anti-inflammatory action."

However, the latest research is from the Department of Molecular Biology at the Daiichi University of Pharmacy in Japan.[12] This research indicates that CBDA inhibits migration of the highly invasive MDA-MB-231 human breast cancer cells. The data now suggests for the first time that CBDA found in raw cannabis offers a real potential in stopping cancer cell migration, including aggressive breast cancers.

If you do have access to sufficient fresh cannabis leaf and wish to see if you can benefit from juicing, then it is recommended that patients juice around 20 freshly picked cannabis leaves per day for at least 45 days of juicing. To counteract the bitterness, patients mix the cannabis juice (1 part) with carrot juice (10 parts) and the juice should be consumed three times daily. This is only realistically possible if you can cultivate your own crop, and unfortunately for most patients, growing several large cannabis plants in the vegetative stage in order to provide yourself with enough fresh leaves for juicing will never be a viable option.

Many patients advise juicing whole, seeded cannabis buds instead of the leaf, and this may have some merit. By using seeded flowers, you are not only benefiting from an increased level of cannabinoid acids, but from the seed content as well. The medical benefits of large doses of acidic cannabinoids have not been subjected to controlled clinical trials, and all of the evidence at this point is anecdotal. Fresh cannabis plant material can harbor a wide range of pathogenic microbes, so anyone with a compromised immune system would be well advised to exercise caution when juicing.

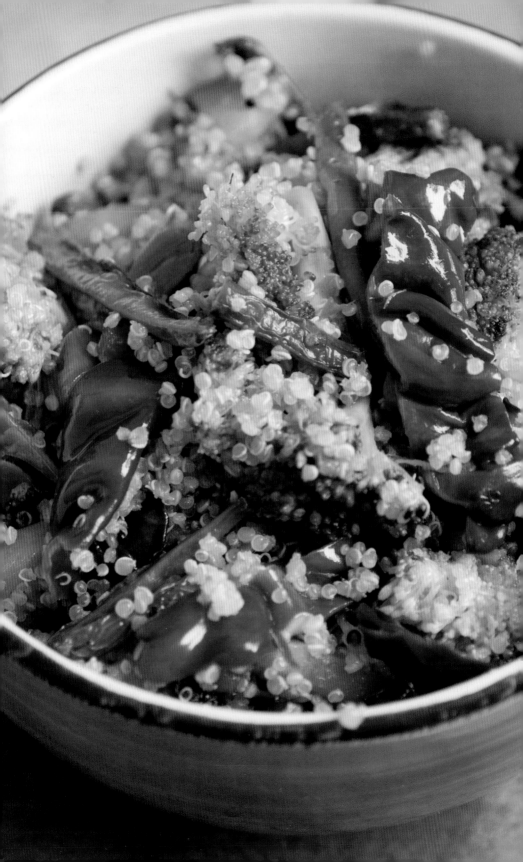

CHAPTER SEVEN

The Cannabis Kitchen

Eating cannabis is an effective delivery method, and the cannabis concentrates and extracts in this chapter will allow you to easily convert any conventional recipe into an effective medicinal or recreational snack or meal. There is little point in preparing a huge, calorie-laden meal and then adding cannabis to it, as the digestive process simply takes too long and diminishes the effects. It is better to prepare simple dishes that are easily digested. In order to convert the active components of cannabis, the plant material still has to be heated when preparing edibles, but the important thing to understand is that, once ingested, it can take between 30 minutes to an hour and a half before the first stages of the high are even noticed. After this, the euphoric state continues to increase. It may then last from four to eight hours, and in some cases, may last even longer and be far more powerful than smoking the same amount. Cannabis edibles can produce a very intense, almost psychedelic experience, particularly if you overdo the amount ingested. It is advisable to experiment with smaller quantities until you are satisfied with the effect produced.

The psychopharmacological effects of ingested cannabis are very different from those experienced after inhaling smoke or vapor into the lungs, as many of the active components in cannabis are altered or destroyed during combustion. When cannabis has been ingested, the peaks of the experience tend to appear in successive waves, and these are far stronger than users

A healthy diet is essential when using medicinal cannabis.

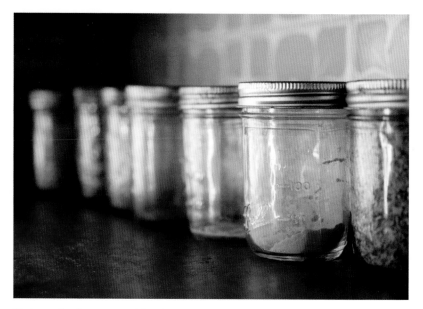

Herbs and spices are nutritional powerhouses.

will experience through smoking, with the effects lasting much longer. This is partly due to enzymes and other fluids in our digestive system that subtly alter the structure of the cannabinoids, but also due to the delayed onset of the effects after ingestion as there is an absence of any immediate sensation which would indicate to the cannabis smoker that enough has been taken. When eaten, some of the THC is metabolized by the liver into 11-Hydroxy-THC, which is four to five times more psychoactive. It is not possible to have a toxic reaction to the ingested cannabis unless you suffer from one of the extremely rare cases of cannabis hyperemesis; however, if you ingest too much you will almost certainly fall into a deep, unconscious sleep, and this could last for over 12 hours. If you are feeling the effects of ingesting too much cannabis, then a tablespoon of honey in warm water can help to reduce the intensity.

As the cannabinoids in cannabis will not dissolve in water, most edibles require some form of extraction method, either into a fat, oil or alcohol medium. Cannabinoids can also be extracted by simmering your plant material in full fat milk as they will readily dissolve into these fats, and this is the method used to prepare the Indian cannabis drink known as bhang. Most cannabis cookery books rely heavily on the use of cannabis butter, which is a very effective method for administering cannabinoids. Canna-flour is ideal for making bread and for use in cakes and pastries.

Cannabis tincture is a concentrated cannabinoid extract dissolved in alcohol that is easily added to meals and drinks, as alcohol solutions are readily assimilated, even in the absence of digestive secretions, and easily absorbed through the stomach lining. Honey and other sugars are also rapidly absorbed into the bloodstream through the intestinal capillaries; however, THC does not dissolve readily in sugars and therefore the degree of absorption is limited. A small quantity of sugar contained within alcohol or an oil-based edible does facilitate absorption, but too much sugar will interfere with the digestion of the cannabinoid loaded fats. Canna-butter or ghee is used for baking and can also be used as a spread, for example on toasted bread or fruit cakes. Canna-infused oils are a useful addition to salad dressing, and they can be used in most recipes as a replacement for butter, particularly if you are lactose intolerant or avoiding dairy products. Heated and ground cannabis buds can also be sprinkled onto cereals or added to savory dishes without any need for preparing a canna-edible dish.

Decarboxylating Cannabis

Freshly harvested cannabis will contain a large amount of THC in the form of tetrahydrocannabinolic acid (THCA). This acid is not psychoactive, but as the

Effect of heating time and temperature on the THC content of n-hexane marijuana extract after heating on the glass surface in an open reactor

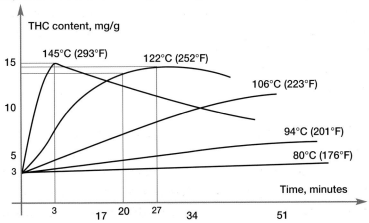

Source: Journal of Chromatography 520 (1990)

plant material dries it converts to active THC by a natural process known as decarboxylation. Most of the acid will convert to THC during a period of up to two years, but by then most of the THC will have oxidized into cannabinol. The heating process is used to speed decarboxylation within the plant material, either in the form of smoking or gentle cooking for edibles. Amino acids have a two-carbon bond. One of these carbons is part of a group called the carboxyl group. The decarboxylating process causes the removal of a carboxyl group within the cannabis material, in order to convert the cannabinoids into substances that will produce a psychoactive effect. The resultant plant material can then be used to make your concentrates.

It is good practice to make your cannabis concentrates as potent as possible as the strong taste of raw cannabis can be quite overpowering, so the more potent the concentrate, the less you require in your recipes. Using concentrates alongside conventional ingredients results in a better-tasting product. For example, if a cake recipe calls for 200 grams of butter, then it is preferable to use 100 grams of your cannabis butter alongside 100 grams of regular butter. To decarboxylate your plant material, take your cannabis bud or trim and spread it evenly on a baking tray or ovenproof plate, then place into an oven set on 223°F (106°C). Don't set the temperature any higher as the additional heat will vaporize the cannabinoids. After 25 minutes, using oven gloves remove the cannabis from the oven and it should be dry and crisp.

Basic Canna-Concentrates: Canna-Flour

Preparation Time: 10 minutes

Equipment: Coffee grinder or food processor.

Ingredients:

■ Any quantity of decarboxylated cannabis material.

Place the decarboxylated plant material into an herb grinder or food processor, and process for a few minutes until finely powdered.

Place a fine sieve over a collection bowl and sift the powder, discarding any stalks or leaf veins.

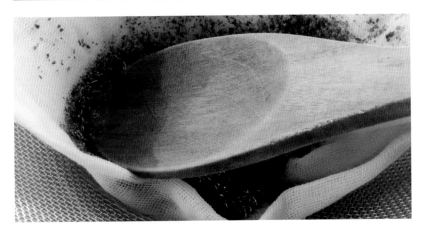

Always strain your cannabutter extremely well.

Bread made solely from canna-flour can have a strong residual flavor for most tastes, and many people find that one part canna-flour to two parts of regular flour is a good combination. The flour is ideal for making bread and pastries and it also makes palatable cookies, but for cakes it is a little heavy, and it is better to use canna-butter instead.

Canna-Butter

Preparation Time: Around 12 hours

Equipment: 1 slow cooker (also known as a crock pot). One French press (also known as a coffee press, coffee plunger or cafetière à piston).

Ingredients:

- 1 pound of unsalted butter
- 2 pints of water and 2 ounces of premium, high-grade cannabis (leaf trimmings are fine to use but not as strong so it is advisable to add 25% more).

Break up your dried cannabis and place this into a slow cooker with the butter and water. Set the temperature to high and once all of the butter has melted, turn the heat setting to low. The addition of the water helps to keep the temperature down, and the additional volume allows for more plant material to be added, particularly if you are using trimmings. As cannabinoids are soluble in fats and oils but not water, they will be absorbed into the butter, so allow the mixture to simmer on a low heat for 4 hours, stirring every 30 minutes. After the allotted time, turn off the heat and allow the mixture to cool.

STEP-BY-STEP Canna-Butter

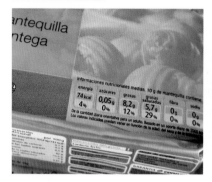

1. Butter.

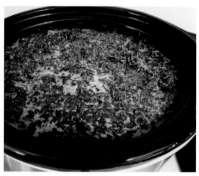

2. Using a crock pot to gently heat the butter and cannabis.

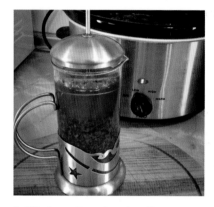

3. Filtering using a french coffee press.

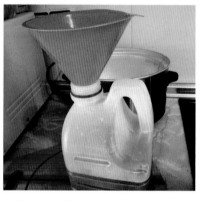

4. Place the filtered butter into a plastic container.

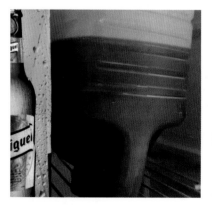

5. Store in the fridge.

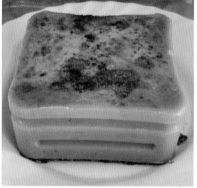

6. Cut the plastic container to remove the set butter.

Once it has cooled (but is still warm), carefully ladle the mixture from the slow cooker into a sieve suspended over a clean pan. Pour boiling water over the plant material in the sieve, and use the back of a large spoon or ladle to expel as much liquid from the vegetable matter as possible. Complete the final filtering process by carefully pouring the butter and water mix into your coffee press, and pushing down on the plunger. It is possible to strain the mixture through muslin or cheesecloth, but it is much easier to use a coffee press. Pour the sieved liquid into a clean plastic bottle for storage and place the container upside down in your refrigerator overnight, ensuring that it is vertical and cannot fall over. When you remove the bottle from the refrigerator the next day, the butter will have solidified.

Hold the plastic bottle containing the solidified canna-butter over a large bowl or washbasin, and slowly unscrew the cap. The water will now flow out, leaving you with the just the canna-butter. Using a box cutter, sharp knife or scissors, carefully cut open the plastic bottle and remove the canna-butter. This can now be cut into 1-ounce (28 grams) portions that can be frozen for long-term storage.

Potency and Dosage Calculator for Canna-Butter

Using 1 pound of butter and 2 ounces of bud will result in the extract from ⅛ of an ounce (3.5 grams) of cannabis per ounce (28 grams) of canna-butter.

Canna-Ghee

Ghee is clarified (purified) butter that originated in Asia and is commonly used in Indian, Bangladeshi, Nepali, Pakistani and Iranian cuisine and ritual. Canna-ghee is made from canna-butter and will keep for many months without the need for refrigeration.

Preparation Time: 1 hour

Equipment: One medium-sized saucepan, a fine sieve or larger sieve with two layers of muslin cloth and one large spoon.

Ingredients:
■ 1 pound of canna-butter.

To convert canna-butter into ghee, you will need to place a quantity into a medium-sized saucepan and cook uncovered on a low to medium heat until all of the butter has melted. Slowly increase the heat until the liquid butter is simmering (but do not allow to boil).

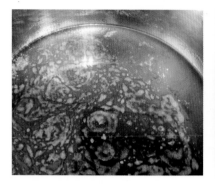

Cannabis simmering in ghee.

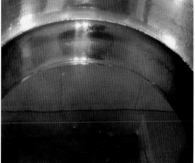

Allow ghee to cool before straining.

Continue cooking whilst stirring occasionally until the butter starts to foam. If you hear a crackling noise, the butter has begun to boil and you should reduce the heat setting. Froth will begin to appear on the surface; remove this with the spoon and discard. Continue this process until no more froth appears, and the ghee becomes a clear golden-yellow liquid, indicating the butter has clarified. Be careful not to overcook the ghee or burn the solids. If the milk solids appear dark in color, or if the liquid ghee turns dark brown, you have overcooked it.

Let the ghee cool for about 20 minutes, and then strain it though a very fine strainer or 2 layers of muslin cloth placed inside a sieve. Make sure all the milk solids are strained out, and repeat the process if needed. Store your canna-ghee in a clean, dry and airtight container. It will keep for over 2 months without the need for refrigeration.

Ghee Potency and Dosage Calculator

Your canna-butter will already contain the extract from ⅛ of an ounce (3.5 grams) of cannabis per ounce of butter (28 grams), and during the production of ghee you can expect to lose as much as 25% of the original volume. This increases the potency of your ghee proportionately but is far from an accurate guide. Just be advised that you will require less ghee than canna-butter when preparing your canna-edibles.

Canna-Infused Oil

This is an edible infusion and not a medical-grade extract; it is not to be confused with medicinal hemp oil, which is extracted from the cannabis flowers using solvents.

Preparation Time: 2 hours

STEP-BY-STEP Cannabis-Infused Oil

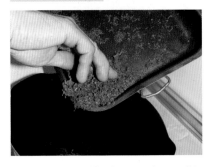

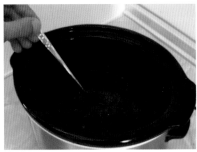

1. Add dried and finely ground cannabis to the oil.

2. Simmer for 2 hours, stirring occasionally.

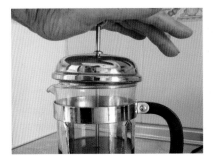

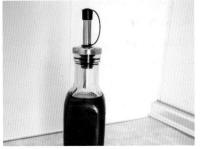

3. Filter the oil using a coffee plunger.

4. Store the oil in its original bottle.

Equipment: 1 slow cooker, a coffee grinder (or food processor), French press and a fine sieve.

Ingredients:

■ 1 quart of vegetable oil (hemp oil, olive oil, coconut oil, sunflower or vegetable oil), 2 ounces of cannabis buds or leaf trimmings.

Place one quart of your chosen oil into your slow cooker. Set the controls to low, and, adding your dried and ground cannabis, simmer for 2 hours, stirring occasionally. Allow to cool, and then carefully ladle the oil from the slow cooker into the coffee plunger. Once filtered, pour the oil back into the original bottle.

This infused cannabis oil can be used in salad dressings, baking or simply drizzled over fresh bread. Rather than using your canna-infused oil as a salad dressing you can use it to make vinaigrette that will liven up any salad. It can also be used in stir fries or as a marinade.

Canna-Infused Vinaigrette

Preparation Time: 5 minutes

Ingredients:

- Any amount of canna-infused oil
- An equal amount of balsamic vinegar
- 2 cloves of finely chopped garlic
- ½ teaspoon dried oregano
- 2 teaspoons mustard (optional)
- salt and pepper to taste

Combine and serve.

Dosage Calculator for Infused Oil

1 quart of oil is equivalent to approximately 64 tablespoons, so if you have used 2 ounces (56 grams) of cannabis buds then four tablespoons will contain the extract from ⅛ of an ounce (3.5 grams) of cannabis.

Green Dragon Rum Infusion

Preparation Time: 30 minutes

Equipment: Coffee grinder, saucepan, small storage jar, cooking thermometer, fine strainer.

Ingredients:

- 2 ounces of rum (white or dark), ⅛ ounce of ground dried cannabis buds.

Finely grind your herbal cannabis, and then add 2 ounces of rum to your storage jar. Place the storage jar into a saucepan of water and simmer for 20 minutes. Maintain the water temperature at around 155°F. Strain the mixture and as with all of these concentrates and edibles store them safely away from children in a refrigerator or cool dark area.

Dosage Calculator for Green Dragon

Taken alone 1 to 2 tablespoons will give you a noticeable effect that can last for several hours.

STEP-BY-STEP	Alcohol Infusion

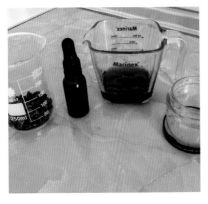

1. Equipment required for alcohol infusion.

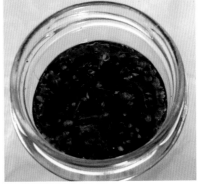

2. Soak the dried cannabis buds in alcohol.

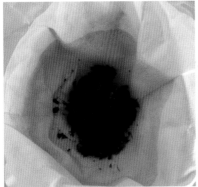

3. Filter the liquid.

4. Store in a dropper bottle.

Easy Canna-Edible Recipes

A Traditional Bhang Preparation

This is an ancient and popular drink in India, made from flowers of the cannabis plant. It has special religious significance during the festivals of Holi, Maha Shivratri and Kali Puja. It is prepared by grinding cannabis buds and mixing them with milk, ghee and spices. The following recipes are taken from *On the Preparation of the Indian Hemp* by W. B. O'Shaughnessy (1843):

"Sidhee, subjee, or bhang [cannabis] is used with water as a drink, which is thus prepared. About three tola weights [35 grams] are well washed with cold water, and rubbed to powder, mixed with black pepper, cucumber and melon seeds, sugar, 30 cl. of milk, and an equal quantity of water. This is considered sufficient to intoxicate a habituated person. Half the quantity is enough for a novice.

This composition is chiefly used by the Mohammeds of the better classes."

A second recipe is also described by O'Shaughnessy:

"The same quantity of sidhee [cannabis] is washed and ground, mixed with black pepper, and a liter of cold water added. This is drunk at one sitting. This is the favorite beverage of the Hindus who practice this vice, especially the Birjobassies, and many of the Rajpootana soldiery. From either of these beverages intoxication will ensue in half an hour. Almost invariably the inebriation is of the most cheerful kind, causing the person to sing and dance, to eat food with great relish, and to see aphrodisiac enjoyments. In persons of quarrelsome disposition it occasions, as might be expected, an exasperation of their natural tendency. The intoxication lasts about three hours, when sleep supervenes. No nausea or sickness of stomach succeeds, nor are the bowels at all affected; next day there is slight giddiness and vascularity of the eyes, but no other symptom worth recording."

Contemporary Bhang Recipe

Preparation Time: 20 minutes

Equipment: Coffee grinder (or food processor), French press, large bowl.

Ingredients:

- 2 cups water
- 1 ounce of decarboxylated marijuana
- 4 cups warm milk
- 2 tablespoons blanched and chopped almonds
- ⅛ teaspoon garam masala (cloves, cinnamon, and cardamom)
- ¼ teaspoon powdered ginger
- 1 teaspoon rosewater
- 1 cup sugar

Bring the water to a rapid boil and pour into a clean receptacle containing your cannabis. Let stand for 10 minutes. Strain the water and cannabis using your coffee press, collect the water and save. Squeeze as much liquid as possible from the cannabis pulp and then, whilst still in the coffee grinder, add two teaspoons of warm milk. Strain the cannabis through your coffee press again and squeeze out as much milk as you can.

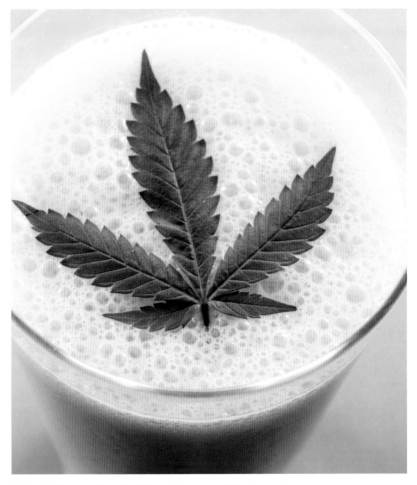

This delicious and healthy Bhang takes only 20 minutes to prepare.

Repeat this process 5 times. Collect all the milk that has been extracted and save. By this time the cannabis will have turned into a pulpy mass. Remove from the coffee press, and add the chopped almonds and some more warm milk. Grind this until a fine paste is formed. Strain and squeeze this paste in your coffee press and collect the extract as before.

Repeat a few more times until all that is left are some fibers and nut meal. Discard the residue. Combine all the liquids that have been collected, including the water the cannabis was brewed in. Add to this the garam masala, dried ginger and rosewater. Add the sugar and remaining milk. Chill and serve immediately.

Hot Buttered Bhang (2 servings)

Preparation Time: 5 minutes

Ingredients:

- 55 grams butter or ghee
- 10 to 15 grams good cannabis tops or leaves
- ¼ liter vodka
- powdered cardamom (optional)
- honey (optional)
- whipped cream (optional)

Melt the butter in a saucepan. Crumble in the cannabis and stir. Continue stirring over medium heat for 1 minute. While the mixture is still hot and sizzling, add the vodka. Be cautious that the hot butter does not make the mixture spatter. It is best to pour in the vodka swiftly.

Continue to boil for 30 seconds or more, stirring all the while. The cardamom may be added during the boiling. The longer you boil, the less alcohol the drink will have. After boiling for desired time strain the liquids. Press the mash with a spoon to remove all the liquids. The effects may be felt in less than 15 minutes.

Quick and Simple Bhang Recipe

Preparation Time: 5 minutes

Ingredients:

- ⅛ ounce unsalted butter
- 2 cups milk
- 4 grams of decarboxylated and ground cannabis
- pinch of cinnamon and/or nutmeg

Melt butter in pan, add ground cannabis, and simmer for 1 minute, then add milk and spices. Simmer gently for a further 3 minutes, then remove from the heat, chill and serve. The bhang can be sweetened with a little honey if required.

Chocolate Brownies Made with Cannabis-Infused Oil

Preparation Time: 45 minutes

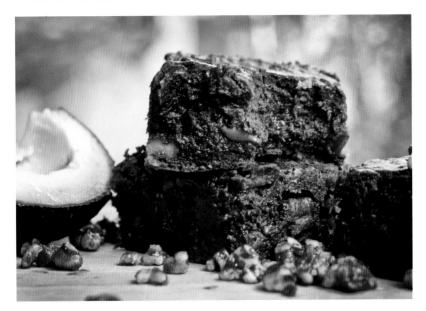

Brownies are a typical choice, but avocado brownies are a healthy alternative.

Ingredients:

- 5 ounces plain chocolate chopped into small pieces
- ½ cup canna-infused oil
- 7.5 ounces (1 cup) of light Muscovado (brown) sugar
- 2 eggs
- 1 teaspoon of vanilla essence
- ½ cup of all-purpose flour
- 1 teaspoon baking powder
- 4 tablespoons of cocoa powder
- 3 ounces (⅓ of a cup) of chopped walnuts or pecan nuts
- 4 tablespoons milk chocolate chips

Preheat oven to 350°F. Lightly grease a shallow 7.5-inch-square cake tin. Melt the plain chocolate in a heat-proof bowl over a saucepan of barely simmering water. Beat the canna-infused oil, sugar, eggs and vanilla essence together in a large bowl. Stir in the melted chocolate and continue to beat well, until evenly mixed and smooth.

Sift the flour and the cocoa powder into the bowl and fold in thoroughly. Stir in the chopped nuts and chocolate chips, tip into the prepared tin and spread evenly to the edges. Bake the mix for 30 to 35 minutes, or until the top is firm and crusty. Cool in the tin before cutting into squares.

You can also substitute one third of the regular organic self-raising flour for canna-flour for a stronger, more rustic-tasting brownie.

Cannabis Chocolate

Preparation Time: 15 minutes

Equipment: A saucepan, a glass bowl and a chocolate mold or ice-cube tray.

Ingredients:
- 1 ounce of decarboxylated and finely ground cannabis buds
- 14 ounces of chocolate (at least 70% cocoa solids).

STEP-BY-STEP Cannabis Chocolate

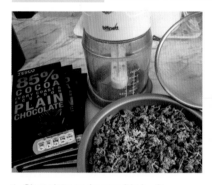

1. Chocolate and cannabis buds.

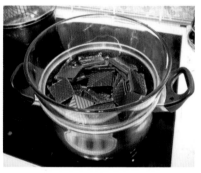

2. Break up chocolate.

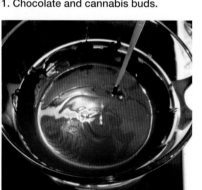

3. Melt over boiling water.

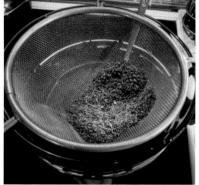

4. Add the cannabis through a sieve.

Place a glass bowl on top of a saucepan containing simmering water (not boiling). Ensure that the water does not come into contact with the bowl as you want to use the steam of the simmering water to gently melt your chocolate.

Break up your chocolate into pieces and place in the bowl. Allow the chocolate to melt slowly and gradually. When your chocolate is fully melted, you can add your ground cannabis and mix thoroughly. Carefully spoon the mix into your chosen mold or ice-cube tray.

When the tray is full, gently raise it up 4 inches and then drop it onto your worktop. This removes any trapped air from within the chocolate and gives a better finished product. Place the mold into a refrigerator and allow it to set. You could wrap your chocolates in foil wrappings, which are available on eBay, to give a professional finish to your chocolates.

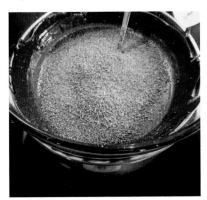

5. Stir in the cannabis gently.

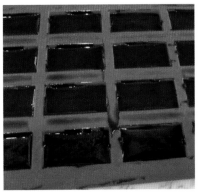

6. Pour the mixture into molds and cool.

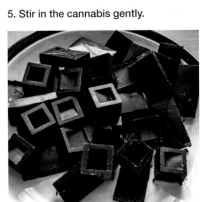

7. Finished canna chocolate.

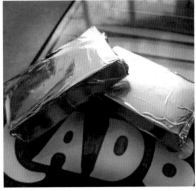

8. Foil wrappers give a professional finish.

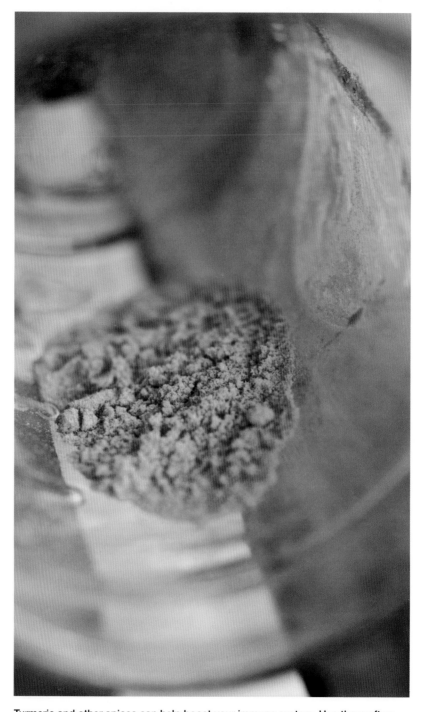

Turmeric and other spices can help boost your immune system. Use them often.

Cannabis Lozenges

Lozenges have been used to administer herbal medicines for hundreds of years and are fairly simple to make at home. As lozenges are dissolved in the mouth the increase in sublingual absorption means your medication enters the bloodstream far more quickly than regular cannabis edibles.

Contemporary Lozenge Recipe

Preparation Time: 15 minutes

Equipment: Large saucepan, sugar thermometer (also referred to as a candy thermometer), lightly oiled ice-cube tray, metal spoon.

Ingredients:

- ½ cup light corn syrup
- ¼ cup white sugar
- ¼ cup canna-butter
- ¼ teaspoon salt
- one sachet or ⅛ cup of powdered drink mix of your choice to add flavor

Combine sugar, salt, corn syrup and butter in a large saucepan and bring to the boil, stirring constantly. Once the mixture is bubbling, lower the heat and continue until your thermometer reads 270°F, before stirring in one sachet of your chosen powdered drink mix. Using a spoon, pour the mixture into your lightly oiled ice-cube tray (only partly fill each section) to make 20 lozenges.

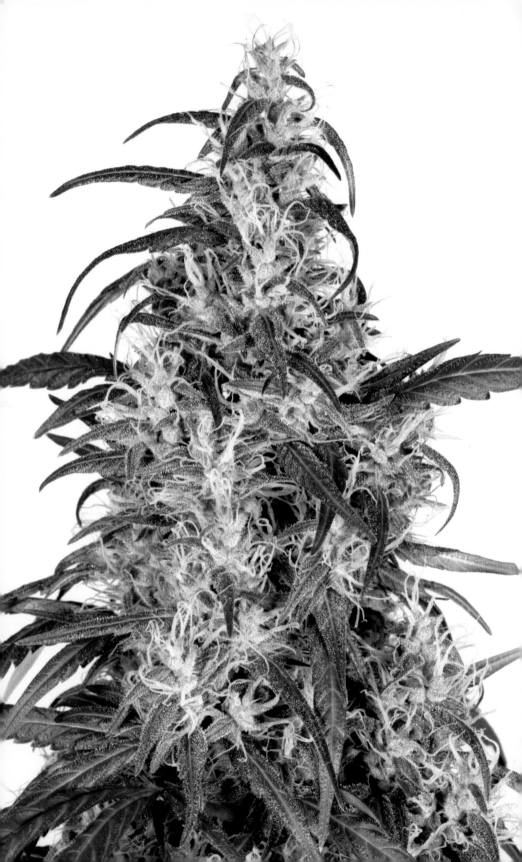

CHAPTER EIGHT

Medicinal Cannabis Growing

It is illegal to grow cannabis in most countries; however, the following information could save your life, and it is disgraceful that cancer sufferers have to make the choice between being a dead law-abiding citizen or a cancer-surviving criminal. The cost of cannabis available on the black market makes the treatment of many of the conditions that can be alleviated or cured through medical cannabis use prohibitively expensive for most patients, and cancer sufferers are particularly badly affected as they require at least a pound of high quality cannabis buds to make an oil extraction. Furthermore, the quality of illicitly produced cannabis can vary considerably and as there is no such thing as quality control in illegal cannabis production, there is no guarantee that the product has not been contaminated with noxious pesticides or chemicals, nor that other substances have not been added to the crop. Adulterated cannabis known as "grit weed" can have anything from sand to silicon sprinkled onto the buds before harvest in an attempt to increase their weight.

In order to benefit from the plant's medicinal properties, the only answer for many patients is to cultivate their own crop. Cultivating cannabis is a fairly straightforward process and only requires a basic understanding of the plant's nutritional and environmental requirements. Cannabis is a hardy plant that grows in diverse and sometimes challenging environments, and it requires no

Sativa-dominant female plant nearing harvest.

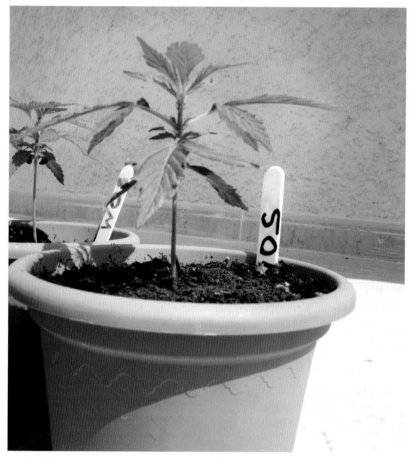

Young seedlings in pots.

specialist knowledge or equipment to produce enough high-quality buds to treat any of the conditions for which it is recommended.

The Basics

There is nothing complicated about growing cannabis. The advice we give here is geared toward producing enough dried cannabis to treat you, using simple techniques and readily available equipment. All cannabis plants, regardless of variety, have the same basic requirements:

- Nutrients and pH in the correct balance.
- Humidity and temperature within the correct range.

- Light of the correct spectrum.
- Water at the correct temperature.
- Air rich in carbon dioxide and well circulated.

Nutrients

These will initially be supplied by your compost mix. Avoid peat and choose a multipurpose loam or organic-based compost. Mix it 50/50 with perlite. Your compost will have enough nutrients within it to sustain plant growth for several weeks depending on the pot size used, after which time you will need to feed the plants. Plant fertilizers have what is known as an N-P-K rating, which refers to the percentages of (N) nitrogen, (P) phosphorus and (K) potassium that the mix contains. During the vegetative stage cannabis uses more nitrogen, whilst during the flowering stage more phosphorous is required. Any compost mix or plant food recommended for tomatoes is fine to use for your crop, but specialist organic "Grow" and "Bloom" fertilizers specifically designed for cannabis are recommended and available online. Do not overfeed your plants–little and often is best–and follow the manufacturer's recommendations. As soil quality can vary enormously, outdoor plants are better cultivated in large pots containing a compost and Perlite mix.

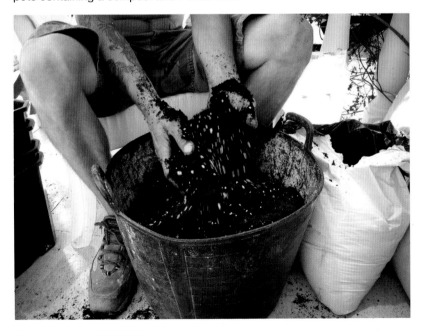

Mixing compost and Perlite.

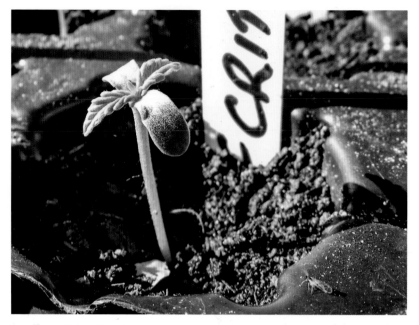

Young seedling with its first set of true leaves emerging, and cotyledons still visible.

pH

Cannabis does not like acidic soil, so the compost mix pH should be between 6.0 and 7.0. You can purchase a simple test probe at your garden store. Compost mixes are very forgiving as they naturally buffer pH themselves. Home remedies to raise or lower pH are:

- pH up: Baking soda. Water plants with ½ teaspoon/gallon.
- pH down: Lemon juice. Water plants with 1 to 2 teaspoons/gallon.

Humidity and Temperature

Humidity is best kept between 40 to 60% during the vegetative phase and 40 to 50% during flowering. The optimal day temperature range for cannabis is 75 to 85°F. The temperature can be allowed to drop during the night. You can buy a combined humidity and thermometer gauge at your garden store.

Light

Sunshine is all you require when growing outside. Indoor growers use artificial light from either HID (high intensity discharge) lamps, specifically HPS (high

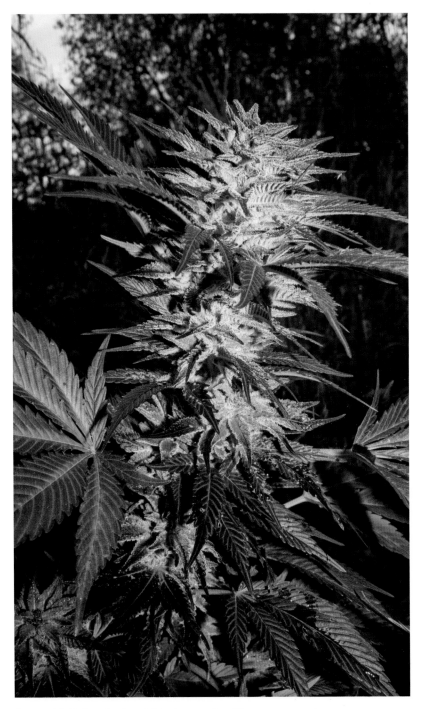

A cannabis indica dominant female, grown outdoors.

pressure sodium) lamps that are suitable for vegetative growth and flowering, or LEDs (light emitting diodes). LEDs are expensive, but do not consume much electricity. Smaller fluorescent and CF (compact fluorescent) lights are ideal for rooting cuttings and starting young seedlings. Lights should be hung as close as possible to the plants without damaging them. Place your hand above your crop to test the heat. If it's too hot for your hand, it is going to harm your crop.

LED lighting recommendations: 1 x 600-watt draw LED lamp will cover a 4 foot x 4 foot area and should return one pound of dried buds, but the cost of these units is high and out of most medical growers' budgets.

HPS lighting recommendations: HPS lamps are inexpensive, particularly low-bay industrial HPS lamps, which are fine to use. You require at least 50 watts of light per one square foot of garden and will get better results using a 600-watt HPS, as that is the most efficient. A simpler guide is:

- 1 x 250-watt HPS illuminates a 2 feet x 2 feet garden
  (4 plants/4 to 5 ounce yield)
- 1 x 400-watt HPS for a 2.5 feet x 2.5 feet garden
  (6 plants/9 to 12 ounce yield)
- 1 x 600-watt HPS for a 4 feet x 4 feet garden
  (9 plants/16 to 18 ounce yield)

Standard Lighting Schedule

From germination until the flowering stage, plants remain under a regime of 18 hours of light and 6 hours of darkness. Flowering is induced by changing the light schedule to 12 hours of light and 12 hours of darkness. Plants receive a minimum of two weeks vegetative growth and eight weeks of flowering.

The Gas Lantern Schedule

Otherwise known as the 12-1 lighting regime, this can save you on average 30 to 50% on your electricity costs, but it also reduces yield. Vegetative growth: 12 hours lights on, 5.5 lights off, 1 hour lights on, 5.5 lights off, and repeat schedule. Flowering: first two weeks 11 hours on, 13 off, the next two weeks 10.5 hours on, 13.5 off, following two weeks 10 hours on, 14 off, following two weeks 9.5 hours on, 14.5 off, and the last two weeks 9 hours on and 15 hours off. Plants receive a minimum of two weeks vegetative growth and eight of flowering.

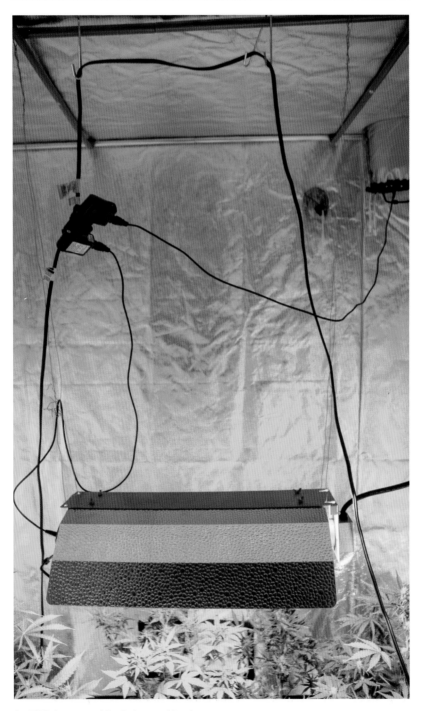

An HPS lamp used for indoor cultivation.

Auto-Flowering Lighting Schedule

There is no requirement to change the lighting cycle when using auto-flowers. The standard practice is to set your schedule to 18 hours on and 6 hours off. Better yields can be obtained at 20 hours on, 4 hours off, but you have a corresponding rise in electricity consumption. The secret with auto-flowering strains is to achieve a balance between yield and energy cost. Plants will trigger flowering automatically after three weeks of vegetative growth with a further five to seven weeks of flowering. Yields will also be less using auto-flowering varieties.

Water Requirements

One of the most common mistakes made by novice growers is to over-water their crop. Warning signs to look out for if you are over-watering include yellowing leaves and slow growth. In order to determine whether a plant needs watering, it is better to lift the pot and gauge its weight. You will soon become accustomed to judging whether or not the plant requires water. Check the pH of your water using an inexpensive aquarium test kit. Some plant feeds are specifically designed for use in hard or soft water areas. One way to determine if your water is hard is to check how it lathers with soap; hard water will have difficulty lathering. In comparison, soft water will lather easily. Rainwater is fine to use.

Air and Carbon Dioxide Requirements

Indoor gardens require that the air temperature be maintained within the ideal range and recirculated. HID lights emit heat so an air extraction system needs to be fitted. You can purchase an "inline" four-inch fan online. This should vent out of the grow space with ducting, and is better purified through a carbon filter to eliminate any pungent odors although this depends on your situation and is not always necessary. Air circulation is best provided using office desk fans blowing over the crop. Carbon dioxide (CO_2) needs to be supplied to the plants so a passive vent (open but with no fan drawing air in) needs to be fitted. There is no requirement to add additional carbon dioxide using CO_2 cylinders. Simply ensure that your extraction system draws in a good supply of fresh air from the outside.

Seeds

High-quality cannabis seeds are readily available for purchase on the Internet; however, it makes good sense to have them delivered to an address where

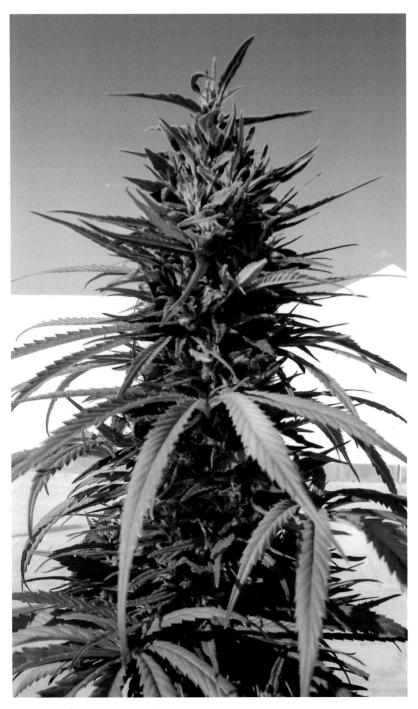

An auto-flowering plant.

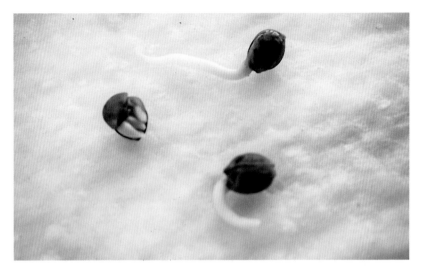

Cannabis seeds sprouting.

no cultivation will take place. Many companies state that they will not ship seeds to the U.S. We have a selection of medical seeds on our website and our supplier ships worldwide, including to the U.S. When germinating regular cannabis seeds you will get a fairly consistent mix of 50% male and 50% female plants. Many medical growers, who have no access to female cuttings from a known, established and reliable source, start their crop with feminized seeds. These seeds are 100% female but produced by a process that used to be referred to as "hermaphroditic breeding." Although feminized seeds are a good way to start an all-female garden, it still takes longer to produce a crop than if you were starting with cuttings taken from a mother plant. It is not advisable to use a plant grown from feminized seeds as a mother plant, and the breeders producing these seeds privately acknowledge this. They are not interested in breeding genetically stable plants that can provide regular cuttings because they want growers to continue purchasing their feminized seeds. It is far better to select a mother plant from regular seeds of known variety and genetics. The mother does not have to be grown from seed, and you can take clones from a clone without any problems.

Germinating Seeds

Many growers germinate seeds by simply planting them into their chosen medium and ensuring they are kept warm and moist. This works well using

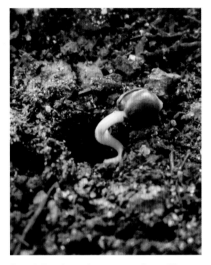
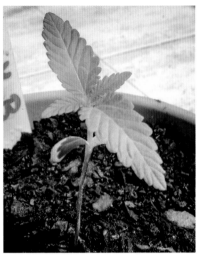

Carefully place the sprouted seedling into fine compost.

A young seedling developing its second set of true leaves.

fine seed compost. Others like to germinate their seeds on saturated tissue paper placed into a shallow dish, but by far the best method is to soak the seeds in a glass of water. After a couple of days the seed casings will split and you will see a root emerging. Remove the seeds and place them into small pots containing fine seed compost. "Damping off" is a fungal infection that attacks the base of the plant stem, killing young seedlings. Give seedlings the best possible start by cleaning all your equipment thoroughly before starting your crop; a dilute 5% bleach solution will kill any fungal spores. Low light levels, low temperatures, high humidity and waterlogged compost all contribute to damping off and should be avoided.

Identifying Cannabis Gender

Even if you are using feminized seeds, it is important to be able to distinguish between male and female plants. When the main flowers first appear they are undifferentiated, which simply means that you can't tell either sex. Soon the male flowers can be recognized by their curved claw shape, followed by the appearance of round and pointed flower buds with five segments. In male flowers, five white petals approximately 3/16 inch (5 millimeters) in length make up the calyx, which is the body of individual flowers. Male petals hang down, and five stamens also approximately 3/16 inch (5 millimeters) in length

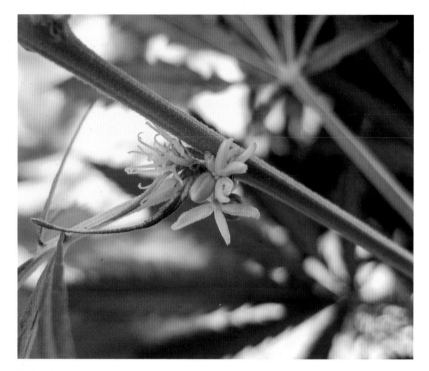

Male cannabis flowers.

emerge. Stamens produce pollen in structures called anthers.

The female calyxes will swell and are easier to distinguish at a younger age than males. The first female calyxes tend to lack paired pistils, which are white pollen-catching structures; however, these soon appear in abundance. As soon as you see two white hairs appear you can confirm your plant is female. Male plants do not produce pistils but some cannabis plants, especially hybrids, produce small nonflowering limbs at each node and these are often confused with male flowers. You must wait until the actual flowers form before positively determining the sex of your plants.

Young seedlings can be forced into flower as soon as they reach three inches (8 centimeters) by placing them into a dark area for 12 hours each day. After two weeks they should show signs of gender, but if they haven't, remove them from the cycle and place them back into the vegetative cycle, as they will still develop small flowers that can be identified. This technique does slow down the plant growth rate and can badly stretch the young plants. It is also suggested that plants treated in this way yield less.

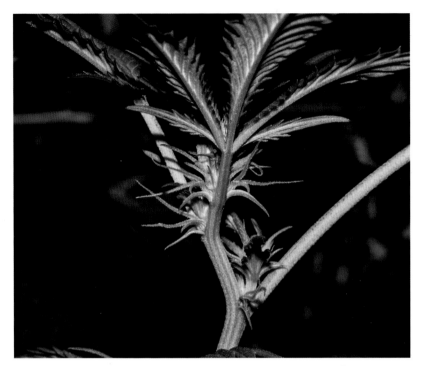

This female plant has just been sexed by the experts at Mandala Seeds in Spain.

Basic Cloning

Cloning, or the taking of cuttings, allows you to cultivate all-female crops with known characteristics. When you take a clone from a female plant, the result-ant offspring will be an exact genetic replica of the mother. The mother is gen-erally kept in a dedicated grow area under a vegetative grow cycle. You can take cuttings from mothers in early flower but it is not advisable.

Equipment: Sharp razor or scissors, rooting gel, clear plastic propagator with lid, fine seed compost, plant mister bottle and small plant pots or Styro-foam cups with drainage holes pierced into the base.

Start by selecting a vigorous growing tip on your chosen female. Ensure that the tip is at least 2 inches (5 centimeters approximately) long, and preferably longer. Cut the tip from the mother plant above the nearest node (the area of a plant's stem from which the leaves grow). The female will go on to produce two fresh growing tips from below the site you have just cut, doubling the number of cuttings that can be taken next time. Re-cut the clone's stem at a slight angle to expose more surface area, and dip the same end into a horticultural rooting

STEP-BY-STEP Cloning

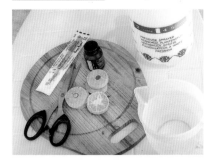

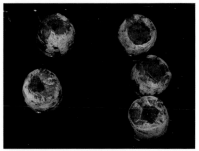

1. Equipment required to successfully clone cannabis plants using peat pellets in this instance.

2. Prepare your peat pellets (Jiffy cubes) by soaking. Jiffy coir pellets are a peat-free alternative.

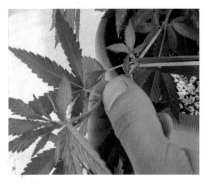

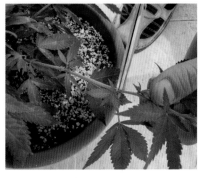

3. Select a vigorous, healthy side shoot from lower down on the plant and cut.

4. Using a sharp pair of scissors or sharp craft knife make a clean cut and remove the side shoot.

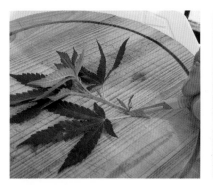

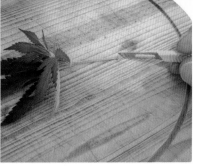

5. Remove excess leaves lower down the side shoots using a sharp scalpel or craft knife.

6. The stem is then cut at a 45° angle to expose more surface area and improve the strike rate.

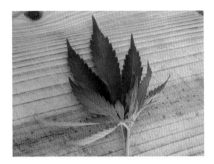

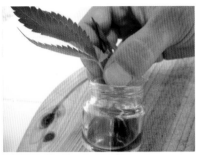

7. A rimmed and cut clone ready for dipping into rooting hormone to help increase the strike rate.

8. Dip the root of the cutting into a rooting hormone. Gels are more effective than powders but you can also use honey.

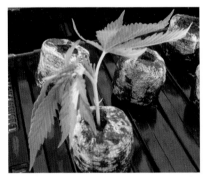

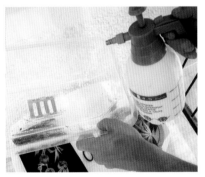

9. Insert the stem of the new clone into a pre-prepared Jiffy cube and place into a plant propagator.

10. Use a mister to give the new clones a fine spray of water at room temperature.

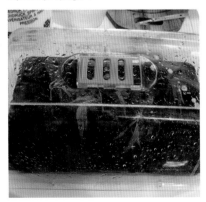

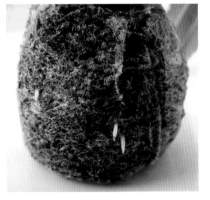

11. A high-sided plant propagator is ideal for keeping the humidity constant for young clones.

12. Newly formed roots can be seen emerging from the sides of the Jiffy cube after 10 to 14 days.

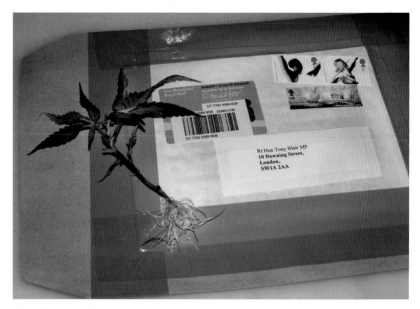

A healthy aero clone.

gel. The clone is then placed into your seed compost and kept in a high-sided propagator. Ensure you have a humid environment for the first few days at least. It is helpful to remove the propagator lid on a daily basis and wipe any excess moisture from the inside using a cloth. Mist the clones daily with a spray bottle for the first few days. Roots should develop within 10 to 14 days.

Pot Sizes

As a general rule you will require one gallon of pot size per foot of plant. Outdoor growers require a minimum of five gallons but most indoor grows will be fine with a three-gallon pot. Starting in smaller pots and transplanting as your indoor garden develops is recommended for several reasons. Most importantly you maximize the use of space and light available, but repotting also helps prevent plants from becoming root-bound, whilst also providing a fresh boost of nutrients and pH buffering.

Vegetative Growth

As soon as your cannabis plants have developed roots, they are ready for the vegetative growing process. Indoor crops are generally left in the vegetative stage for between two weeks to a month before flowering is induced by switching the light cycle.

During the vegetative growth stage, it is advisable to either pinch out the main growing tip or train the plants to produce a compact, higher yielding crop. Lower branches that receive less light and will only produce sparse buds should also be removed. When the growing tip is removed from the cannabis plant's main stem two more shoots will grow from the nodes beneath the cut and this also encourages more growth on the lower branches. Super-cropping is similar to pinching out the main growing tips, but the tip is not removed. This allows the main cola or bud to continue to grow. Crush the innermost part of the main stem below the main cola with your index finger and thumb, ensuring you don't damage the hard outer layer of the stem. This should be done no more than once a week. Crushing this inner part of the stem causes it to become thicker and lower branches increase their growth. Similar results can be achieved by bending the main stem or tying it down. Mesh can be stretched horizontally over the crop and the tops bent to grow beneath it; in this way you increase the light the buds receive. Outdoor gardeners should also employ these training techniques to keep their plants short and bushy.

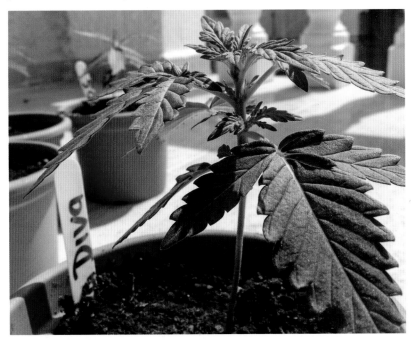

A healthy young seedling in early vegetative growth.

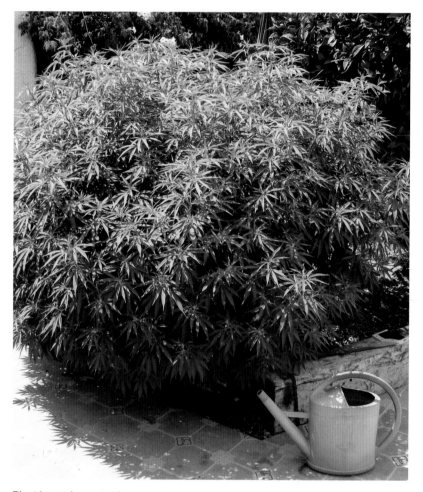

Plant in veg in my garden.

Flowering

After two weeks, or when plants are around 8 to 12 inches tall with good stem development, indoor growers should switch the light cycle to induce flowering. The plants will stretch out slightly as they begin to bloom, but after two weeks they will settle down and concentrate on flower production. Your fertilizer should be changed to a "bloom" formulation, and you should cease all super-cropping techniques. Unless using auto-flowering strains, outdoor growers are dependent on the change in season but can induce flowering earlier by covering plants for 12 hours out of 24. Don't interrupt your light cycles and ensure that no unwanted light is entering your indoor garden as this will disrupt flowering.

Harvesting

After eight weeks of the flowering regime, predominantly cannabis indica varieties will be ready to harvest. Predominantly cannabis sativa varieties may take one to two weeks longer. The seed suppliers will advise you on flowering times. The buds should be sticky and covered with translucent resin, and 50% of the white pistils should have turned brown. Cut the plants at the stem and hang them in a dark area at room temperature. They will dry in around 10 to 14 days. Don't try to speed this process up by applying heat. It is better to be patient and let this process occur naturally. If you are making oil there is no requirement to wait this long for the plants to dry. The main purpose of slow drying is to remove chlorophyll to improve the taste of the cannabis buds.

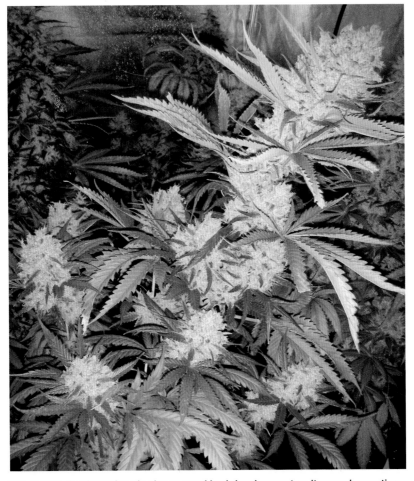

This indica-dominant female shows good bud development as it nears harvesting.

Curing

The curing process breaks down chlorophyll even more and improves flavor in the finished product. We would recommend a minimum of two weeks curing, but the longer the buds are left, the better they will be. Place the dried buds loosely into airtight glass jars in a cool, dark area. The jars should be opened once a day and the buds checked to ensure they are not sweating too much. If they are, they should be removed and further dried. After one week to ten days, the airing process is reduced to a weekly check. Failure to vent the jars will cause moisture buildup and mold will develop, ruining your harvest. If you are making the buds into oil then this process is not required.

The 12-Week Medical Grow

This system will produce enough dried cannabis buds to enable patients to make sufficient cannabis oil for a three-month treatment, which is the recommended dosage for cancer sufferers.

Equipment: 9 feminized cannabis indica–dominant seeds, one 4-foot-square grow tent, one 600-watt High Pressure Sodium lamp, nutrients, compost, Perlite, nine 3-gallon pots, one 4-inch inline fan, one 4-inch desk fan, 4-inch ducting, one time-switch capable of carrying a 600-watt load, one carbon filter (optional).

Grow tents are easy to set up and come with vent sleeves and hanging straps fitted as standard, and they can be purchased cheaply on eBay. Fit the extraction fan and any ducting at the top of the tent with the light hanging beneath it and fitted to your heavy-duty timer. Hang the desk fan so it can be directed over the plants. Germinate your seedlings and place them into the pots. Your seedlings will require three to four weeks in the vegetative stage from germination. After this, begin the flowering cycle. It is recommended that you use the standard 18 hours vegetative growth/12 hours flowering lighting regime for this. After eight weeks in the flowering cycle, you can harvest. After drying, the crop can then be processed into cannabis oil, further cured for vaporizing or used for edibles and drinks.

Advice for Disabled Growers

It is always advisable to have help from your caregiver when setting up, not only for assembling the system, but also for filling the pots with the compost mix. If you have trouble bending, the grow tent can be raised providing there

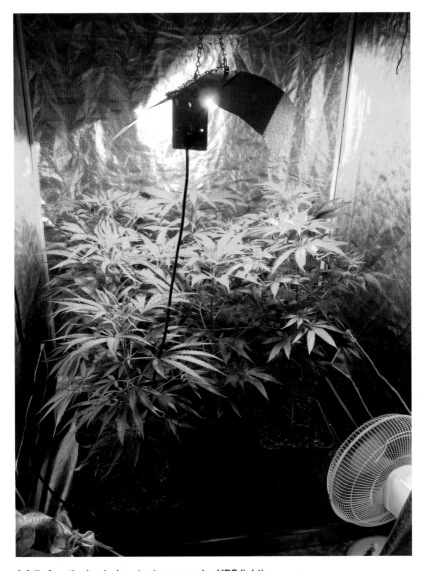

A fully functioning indoor tent grow under HPS lighting.

is enough clearance between the top of the tent and your ceiling.

Many disabled and wheelchair users find it easier to set up what is known as a "lazy Susan." This is basically a rotating base that the plants are grown on. These are constructed using a heavy-duty lazy Susan bearing, available online. The bearing needs to be fitted centrally to a plywood base that sits in the bottom of the tent. The rotating top that the plants will sit on can be either plywood or a heavy mesh, but it needs to be cut to give clearance when rotated. This makes tending and watering the plants far easier.

Blind users find the lazy Susan particularly effective and use talking scales to weigh the pots so that the crop isn't over-watered. Many blind growers also place a graduated bamboo cane into each pot to help gauge the height of their individual plants.

Watering can become a problem for many disabled users who have trouble lifting, so most impaired growers use a pressure sprayer with a hose or lance attachment. If you can lift, it is better to use a small and lightweight, well-balanced plastic watering can with a long narrow spout for reaching into your pots. There are designs available that incorporate a push button at the top of the handle to control the flow of water from the spout, and where the filling hole is covered by a sliding cover to prevent spillage.

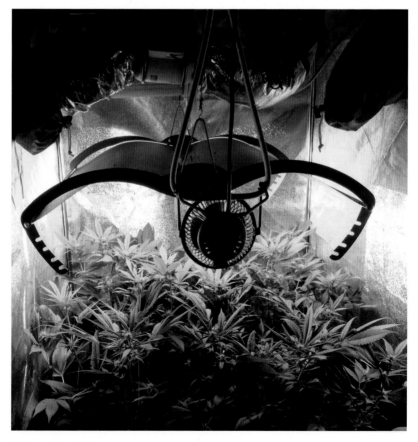

A view of the HPS lamps in this indoor grow.

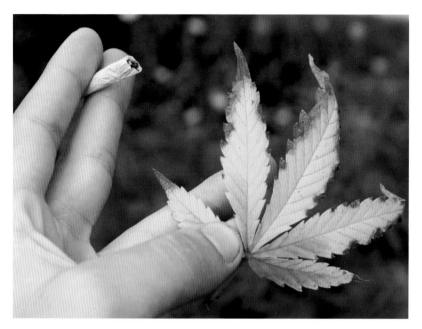

This leaf demonstrates nutrient burn and imbalance in the plant.

Troubleshooting

The worst problem you may get will be insect attacks, and these are easily treated by spraying. As a general rule, it is better to only use pesticides labeled as safe for food crops. Pyrethrins are organic neurotoxins that attack the nervous systems of all insects. When used in smaller doses they have an insect repellent effect. Spider mites are the most damaging pest attack you can suffer but they can be treated using either Neem oil or a specialist spray you can easily source online. Signs of spider mite infestation are seen on the leaves, which will appear speckled as the pests feed on the underside of the leaf. If you have a serious attack, you may see small webs and tiny spider-like insects crawling over the plant.

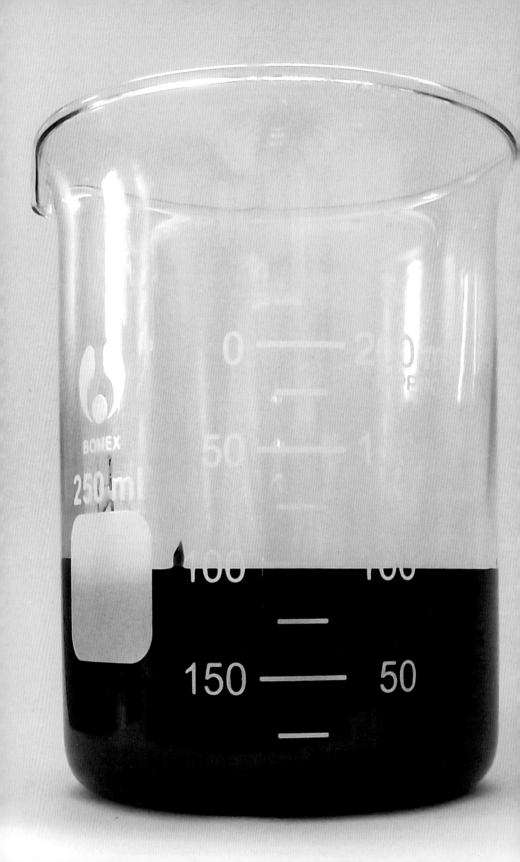

CHAPTER NINE

Frequently Asked Questions

Q: What is the difference between hemp seed oil and cannabis oil?

A: Cannabis oil is a concentrated extract of cannabinoids made from the buds of the illegal drug varieties. Hemp seed oil is made from pressing the oil from seeds of the non-psychoactive commercial hemp plant.

Q: Which cannabis varieties are recommended for making medical cannabis oil?

A: That very much depends on what you want the oil to achieve. The condition you need to treat will determine which variety you choose, depending on whether you require high THC or CBD content. Oil made from a plant that has 50/50 THC and CBD will produce oil with the same cannabinoid profile.

Q: What is the maximum dose of cannabis oil you should take in a 24-hour period?

A: If you are taking it to relieve symptoms then consume as much as you require. The consensus regarding cancer treatment is a minimum of a gram per day.

Q: Is it better to take the oil just before bedtime or do you suggest spreading the dose throughout the day?

A: It is preferable to take the dose throughout the day, but some people prefer to take their daily dose before bedtime.

....

Freshly prepared Bud Buddies 1:1 CBD:THC cannabis oil extraction for medical use.

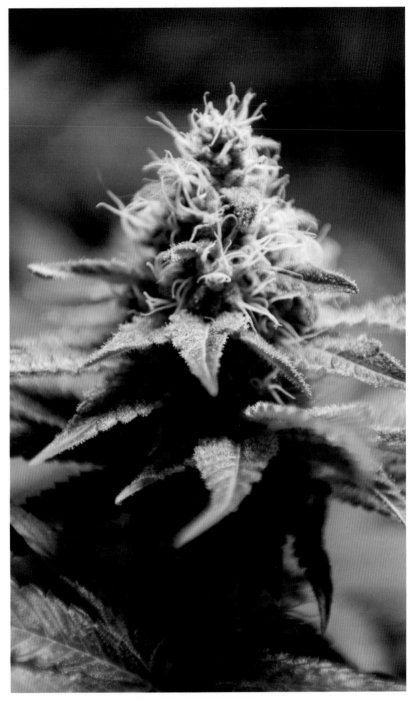

Female flowering.

Q: I have just started on a three-month oil treatment for cancer; when will I become more tolerant to the oil and feel less sleepy?

A: Sleep is an important part of the curing process, but as your dosage increases so should your tolerance.

Q: What is meant by a "maintenance dose," and what dosage is recommended?

A: The dose varies between 0.1 and 0.3 grams per day, generally administered by cancer patients who have taken a full course of oil previously.

Q: Is the evidence that cannabis oil cures cancer purely anecdotal or have there been medical trials?

A: So far all the scientific studies concerning cannabis have been carried out in laboratories, and they have shown conclusively that cannabinoids can kill cancer cells.

Q: How long does it take to grow enough cannabis to make sufficient oil to treat cancer?

A: A 4-foot-square area can provide a pound of cannabis every four months.

Q: Do you treat skin cancer with cannabis ointment, or do you need to complete a three-month oil ingestion treatment as well?

A: Do both if possible, however the consensus is that a topical application is best.

Q: Is it safe to treat children with cannabis oil?

A: Cannabis has very low toxicity and there is no medical reason why it cannot be administered, although obviously the dosage will be less.

Q: Can you make cannabis oil from seeded female flowers?

A: Yes, but bear in mind that seeded cannabis bud has less than half the cannabinoid content of unseeded sensimilla.

Q: What is the best method for storing cannabis oil?

A: Keep it in your refrigerator but make sure that it cannot be accessed by children.

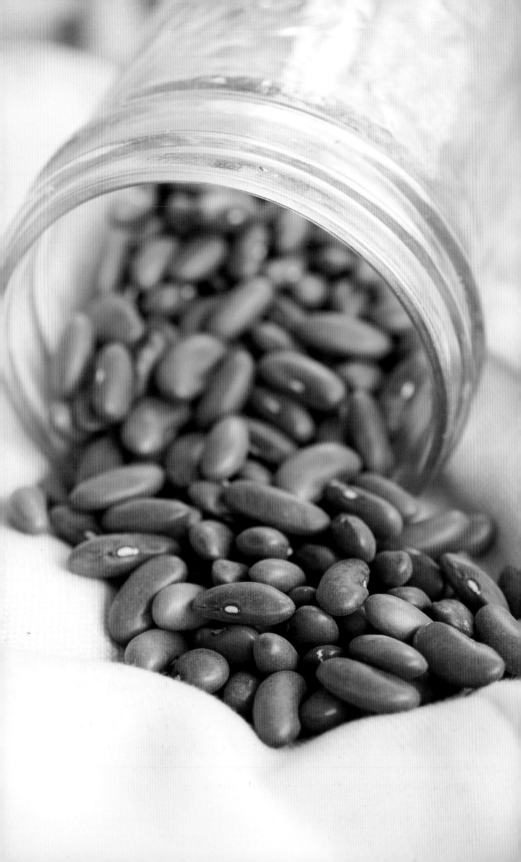

Cancer-Fighting Foods

The best diet for fighting cancer should include unprocessed, predominantly plant-based foods, which includes a variety of vegetables, fruits, whole grains, nuts and beans. Fiber, folate and carotenoids all contribute to the cancer-fighting ability of these foods. Fiber in any form decreases the risk of colorectal cancer, and pancreatic cancer risk is lessened with adequate intake of folate. Try to eat your vegetables either raw or lightly steamed, and choose organic produce whenever possible. Eating red meat substantially raises the risk of cancer or heart disease death; data collected over 28 years reveals a striking link, and it is recommended that you choose fish or poultry instead. Hemp seed should be included in your diet and can replace meat or fish proteins.

Studies have suggested that dairy products may be linked to increased risk for prostate cancer, testicular cancer and possibly for ovarian and breast cancers.[1] Dairy-product consumption increases levels of insulin-like growth factor I (IGF-1) in the bloodstream. IGF-1 is a potent stimulus for cancer cell growth, so it is advisable to either eliminate or at least reduce consumption. The following foods can help inhibit cancer cell growth and are recommended:

Avocados are rich in glutathione, a powerful antioxidant that attacks free radicals in the body by blocking intestinal absorption of certain fats.

Beans, lentils and peas are high in fiber and have components that inhibit cancer reproduction in laboratory studies. The phytochemicals, saponin,

Legumes are low in fat but high in protein, fiber, and nutrients.

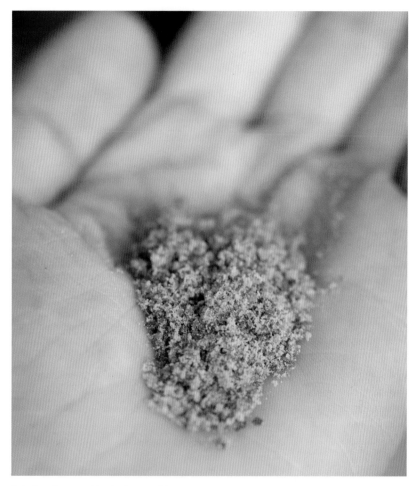

Dried and ground herbal cannabis.

protease inhibitors and phytic acid appear to protect cells from damage.

Broccoli, Brussels sprouts, cabbage and cauliflower contain indole-3-carbinol that helps combat breast cancer by converting a cancer-promoting estrogen into a more protective variety. Broccoli and Brussels sprouts also have the phytochemical sulforaphane, a product of glucoraphanin that is believed to aid in preventing colon and rectal cancer. Broccoli, cauliflower, kale, Brussels sprouts and cabbage contain two antioxidants, lutein and zeaxanthin, that may help decrease prostate and other cancers.

Chili peppers contain capsaicin, which may neutralize certain cancer-causing substances (nitrosamines) and help prevent stomach cancers.

Dandelion Tea: Research indicates that dandelion root extract forces a very aggressive and drug-resistant type of blood cancer cell, known as chronic monocytic myeloid leukemia, to essentially commit suicide, a process called apoptosis. Repeated treatment with low dose dandelion root extract is said to be effective in killing cancerous cells, whilst leaving healthy cells undamaged.

Flax contains lignans, which may have an antioxidant effect and block or suppress cancerous changes. Flax is also high in omega-3 fatty acids, which are thought to protect against colon cancer and heart disease.

Garlic has immune-enhancing allium compounds (dialyl sultides) that appear to increase the activity of immune cells that fight cancer and indirectly help break down cancer-causing substances. These substances also help block carcinogens from entering cells and slow tumor development. Garlic can reduce risk of stomach cancer by half and colorectal cancer by two-thirds when compared to those who eat little or no garlic. The more garlic consumed, the less the risk of these cancers.

Grapes (red) contain bioflavonoids, powerful antioxidants that work as cancer preventatives. Grapes are also a rich source of resveratrol, which inhibits the enzymes that can stimulate cancer-cell growth and suppress immune response. They also contain ellagic acid, a compound that blocks enzymes that are necessary for cancer cells to develop–this appears to help slow the growth of tumors.

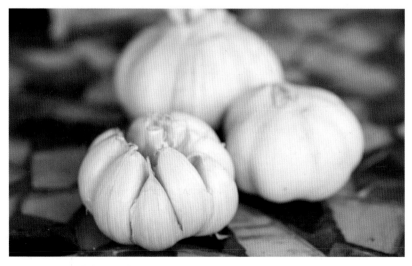

Recent evidence-based research suggests garlic may be effective against some diseases.

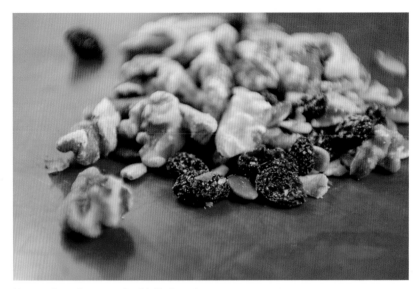

Nuts and seeds are packed full of nutrients.

Hemp Seed and hemp seed oil are known to have anticancer, anti-inflammatory effects and improve the body's ability to respond to insulin.

Kale has indoles, which are nitrogen compounds that may help stop the conversion of certain lesions to cancerous cells in estrogen-sensitive tissues. In addition, isothiocyanates, phytochemicals found in kale, are thought to suppress tumor growth and block cancer-causing substances from reaching their targets. Kale, spinach, collard greens, mustard greens, romaine lettuce, leaf lettuce and swiss chard are all common, dark-green leafy vegetables. The carotenoids in green leafy vegetables, also known as leutein and zeozanthan, act as antioxidants throughout the body.

Mushrooms appear to help the body fight cancer and build the immune system, mainly shiitake, maitake, reishi, Agaricus blazei Murill, and Coriolus Versicolor. These mushrooms contain polysaccharides, especially Lentinan, which are powerful compounds that help in building immunity. They are a source of Beta Glucan. They also have a protein called lectin, which attacks cancerous cells and prevents them from multiplying. They also contain Thioproline. These mushrooms can also stimulate the production of interferon in the body.

Nuts contain the antioxidants quercetin and campferol that may suppress the growth of cancers. Brazil nut contains 80 micrograms of selenium, which

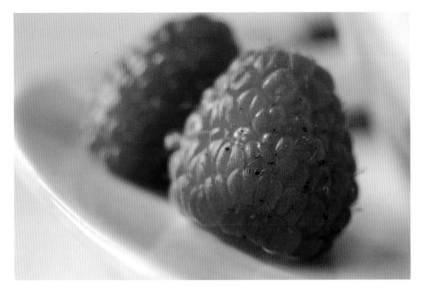

Berries are loaded with antioxidants, protecting your body against inflammation and free radical molecules that can damage cells and organs.

is important for those with prostate cancer.

Oranges and other citrus fruits contain monoterpenes, believed to help prevent cancer by sweeping carcinogens out of the body. Some studies show that grapefruit may inhibit the proliferation of breast-cancer cells in vitro. Oranges and lemons contain limonene, which stimulates cancer-killing immune cells.

Raspberries contain many vitamins, minerals, plant compounds and antioxidants known as anthocyanins, all of which may protect against cancer. According to a recent research study reported by Cancer Research, rats fed diets of 5% to 10% black raspberries saw the number of esophageal tumors decrease. Research reported in the journal *Nutrition and Cancer* in May 2002 shows black raspberries may also thwart colon cancer. Black raspberries are rich in antioxidants, thought to have even more cancer-preventing properties than blueberries and strawberries. Berries are considered good sources of vitamin C, fiber, ellagic acid and other phytochemicals. The American Institute for Cancer Research (AICR) states that ellagic acid is a phytochemical that has antioxidant powers, decreases carcinogens and slows reproduction of cancer cells.

Sweet Potatoes (Yams) contain many anticancer properties, including beta-carotene, which may protect DNA in the cell nucleus from cancer-causing chemicals outside the nuclear membrane.

Teas: Green tea and black tea contain certain antioxidants known as polyphenols (catechins), which appear to prevent cancer cells from dividing. Green tea is rated as the most effective, followed by the more common black tea; however, herbal teas do not show this benefit. According to a report in the July 2001 issue of the *Journal of Cellular Biochemistry*, the polyphenols that are abundant in green tea, red wine and olive oil, may protect against various types of cancer. Dry green tea leaves, which are about 40% polyphenols by weight, may also reduce the risk of cancer of the stomach, lung, colon, rectum, liver and pancreas. AICR reports green tea has the highest concentration of catechins, which have shown potential for preventing cancer cell development in laboratory studies. Population studies show that groups of people who consume high amounts of green tea have lower incidence of bladder, colon, stomach, pancreatic and esophageal cancers.

Tomatoes contain lycopene, an antioxidant that attacks roaming oxygen molecules, known as free radicals, which are suspected of triggering cancer. It appears that the hotter the weather, the more lycopene tomatoes produce. Watermelons, carrots and red peppers also contain these substances, but in lesser quantities. Scientists in Israel have shown that lycopene can kill mouth cancer cells, and an increased intake of lycopene has already been linked to a reduced risk of breast, prostate, pancreas and colorectal cancer.

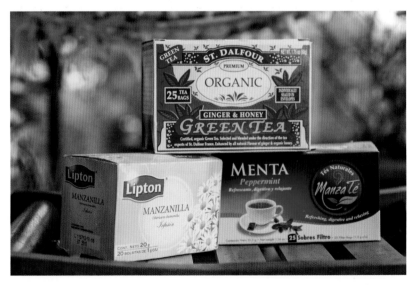

Tea is derived from a particular plant (Camellia sinensis) and includes only four varieties. Herbal teas are technically not teas but an infusion.

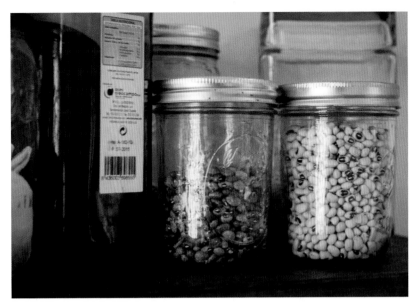

A variety of grains, spices, pulses, and legumes will help you stay healthy.

Turmeric (curcumin) is a polyphenol from the turmeric plant. It has a variety of properties that include antioxidant, analgesic, anti-inflammatory and antiseptic action. It has also been shown to fight cancer by influencing mutagenesis, oncogene expression, cell cycle regulation, apoptosis, tumorigenesis and metastasis. Turmeric has been traditionally used in India as a disinfectant and treatment for laryngitis, bronchitis, and diabetes. It is responsible for the yellow color of Indian curry and American mustard. Curcumin, which has powerful antioxidant and anti-inflammatory properties, is the most active constituent of turmeric and has been shown to limit cell growth in multiple cancers, and in addition, curcumin affects a variety of growth-factor receptors and cell-adhesion molecules involved in tumor growth, angiogenesis and metastasis.

Whole grains contain fiber, which protects against colorectal cancer. Whole grains are also sources of antioxidants, lignans and saponins. These components have shown cancer-fighting properties.

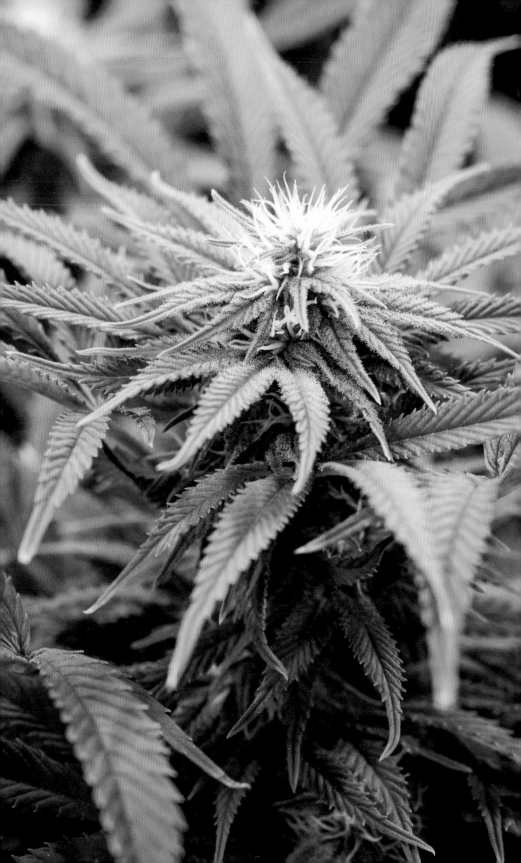

Marijuana Legal Issues

Currently, sick people are being arrested and punished for using medical cannabis when the purpose of law in any democratic country is first and foremost to protect members of its society from harm. Common law (also known as case law or precedent) originated in England in the Middle Ages, and it is implemented in most former colonies of the British Empire, including the United States of America and Canada. English law still provides the basis for many American legal traditions and policies, although it has no superseding jurisdiction. The essence of English common law is that it is upheld by judges sitting in courts, applying common sense and their knowledge of legal precedent to the facts of the case before them. The laws in place should be fair, just and reasonable, with any punishments proportionate to the given crime and based on sensible decisions made by compassionate judges.

Individuals needing to use cannabis to cure illness are some of the most vulnerable in society and the very people that the law was designed to protect. The prohibition of cannabis can in no way be considered fair, just or reasonable. The system of law designed to protect the weakest in society was, and still is, being manipulated by powerful individuals with a purely commercial agenda. Every argument that was put forward to ensure cannabis became illegal has been proven to be false and fraudulent. In essence, the prohibition of cannabis was a corrupt venture, and therefore an illegal undertaking. Furthermore, any

....

White pistils are evident on this maturing female plant.

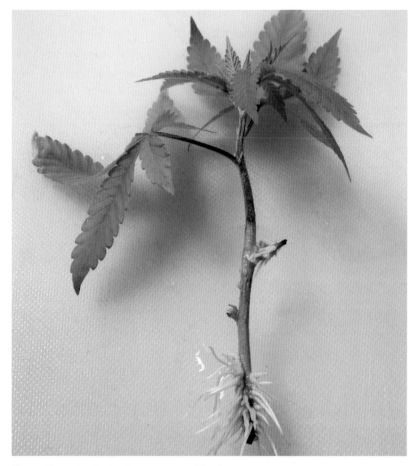

The roots are beginning to emerge on this clone.

person or persons who continue to sustain the criminalization of cannabis are themselves party to this very same corrupt and illegal act.

If you are arrested for any cannabis-related offense, try to stay calm and remember that you do not have to say anything to the police officers. You should not be intimidated into answering questions until you have spoken to a legal adviser. Give only your name, address and telephone number, and your immediate family and employer's numbers if asked. Do not resist arrest, even if you are innocent, as you will be charged with resisting arrest and they may possibly hurt you.

Do not regard the arresting officers as people who are there to help you, regardless of how they speak to you; it is the police officer's duty to get you to incriminate yourself. Anything you say can and will be later used against you in any possible court proceedings.

Do not speak to anyone apart from your legal adviser. If you're arrested with somebody else do not talk to them about the incident. Police vehicles and holding cells are equipped to make video or audio recordings. You have a right to make one phone call but the telephone you use will also be equipped to make an audio recording of your conversation. You have the right not to incriminate yourself. It is the responsibility of the police to prove the charge against you. Warnings regarding the right not to incriminate yourself originated in England in 1912, when the Judges Rules were introduced. These stated that:

"When a police member has admissible evidence to suspect a person of an offense and wishes to question that suspect about the offense, the officer should first caution the person that he is entitled to remain silent."

The giving of this caution in England does not require a suspect to confirm that they understand the caution. Furthermore, the invoking of this right to silence does not prohibit officers from asking further questions. This is not the case in the U.S., where the police cannot interrogate a suspect further unless they waive their right.

Miranda Rights in the U.S.

A Miranda warning is a criminal procedure rule that law enforcement must make in order to protect you from a violation of your Fifth Amendment right against induced self-incrimination. However, in the case of Berghuis v. Thompkins, the Court held that unless a suspect actually states that he is relying on this right, his subsequent voluntary statements can be used in court and police can continue to interrogate the said person. The Fifth Amendment right is the right to remain silent, the right to refuse to answer questions or to otherwise communicate information. Therefore, before any interview takes place the suspect must be advised:

- They have the right to remain silent. Anything the suspect says can be used against them.
- They have the right to have an attorney present before and during the questioning.
- They have the right, if they can't afford an attorney, to have a attorney appointed at public expense to represent them before and during the questioning.

Canada

Equivalent rights exist in Canada consistent with the Charter of Rights and Freedoms. The right to silence is protected under section 7 and section 11(c). The accused may not be compelled as a witness against themselves in criminal proceedings, and therefore only voluntary statements made to police are admissible as evidence. Under the Charter, an arrested person also has the right:

- To be informed promptly of the reasons.
- To retain and instruct counsel without delay and be informed of that right .
- To have the validity of the detention determined by way of habeas corpus and to be released if the detention is not lawful.

European Union

Known as The Reding Rights, those suspected of a criminal offense must receive information about their basic rights during criminal proceedings. These are that they have the right:

- To a lawyer.
- To be informed of the charge.
- To interpretation and translation for those who do not understand the language of the proceedings.
- To remain silent and to be brought promptly before a court following arrest.

They are also informed that:

- They will be given a letter spelling out their rights in writing.
- The letter of rights will be easy to understand, without legal jargon.
- It will be made available in a language the suspect understands.
- It will contain practical details about the person's rights.

Know Your Rights

Habeous corpus was conceived to protect against tyranny and the abuse of the judicial system and is Latin for "you may have the body." It is a writ that requires a person detained by the authorities be brought before a court of law so that the legality of the detention may be examined. The act was passed by the English Parliament in 1679, but the first recorded use of the principle was

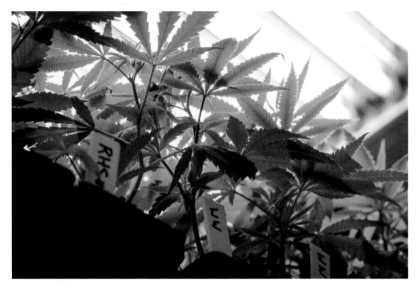

Young plants developing under fluorescent lighting.

in 1305. However, other writs with the same effect appear to precede the English Magna Carta of 1215. Although rarely used nowadays, it can be demanded by anyone who believes they are unlawfully detained and without it you can be imprisoned indefinitely without trial. Habeas corpus rights have been gradually eroded and weakened for over a decade now and the U.S. Patriot Act is just one of the latest efforts to chip away at it.

Samuel R. Caldwell was the first person convicted of selling cannabis under the Marijuana Tax Act of 1937. On the very same day the Marijuana Tax Stamp Act was enacted (Oct. 2, 1937) the FBI and Denver, Colorado police raided the Lexington Hotel and arrested Samuel R. Caldwell, 58, an unemployed laborer and his alleged customer. Caldwell became the first ever cannabis seller convicted under U.S. federal law. His customer was found guilty of possession. Samuel R. Caldwell sold three cannabis cigarettes, and was sentenced to 4 years of hard labor at Leavenworth Penitentiary, in addition to a $1,000 fine. Caldwell was incarcerated in 1937, at age 58, and released in 1940 at age 60. He died one year after his release.

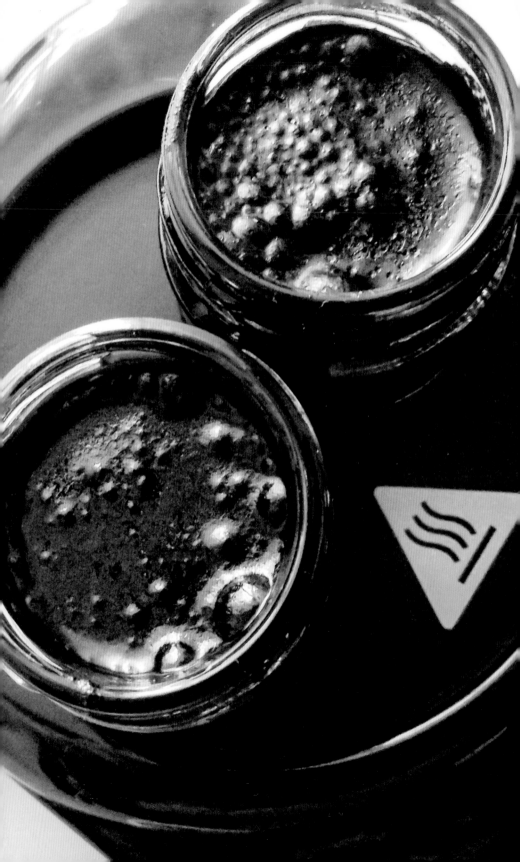

Standardized Medication

If you are making cannabis oil yourself to treat any of the medical conditions that we have detailed in this book, have selected a good quality strain and have carefully followed the instructions given, then your oil should be of sufficient quality to treat the most serious of conditions. This section is designed to help those who wish to learn more advanced techniques for making cannabis oil preparations.

Once you have decided on the cannabinoid profile you require, for example either a high THC or CBD content, and have grown, then processed your selected strain of plants into oil, then the next step in standardizing the medication you are producing is to have your oil laboratory-tested to give you an analysis of the cannabinoid content. When you know the specific percentages of cannabinoids contained in your oil you can accurately calculate the dosage of any medical preparations you make. This is useful when producing capsules and suppositories and allows you to produce medications of varying strengths. This is particularly important when treating children and the elderly as you can moderate the dosage required. There are many companies who will test your oil and the cost is dependent on the method you require them to use. There are three types of test a laboratory can carry out; however, only HPLC will identify how successful your decarboxylation has been and identify phytocannabinoids, GC is not accurate enough.

....

Evaporating on a hot plate.

Gas Chromatography (GC)

Gas chromatography involves the oil sample being vaporized and injected onto the head of a chromatographic column where it can be analyzed. The sample is transported through the column by a flow of chemically inert gas. Commonly used gases include nitrogen, helium, argon and carbon dioxide. The carrier gas system also contains a molecular sieve to remove water and other impurities. This is a common type of chromatography used in analytical chemistry for separating and analyzing compounds that can be vaporized without decomposition. This is the simplest test you can have carried out on your oil and subsequently the least expensive. The results will give you an overall cannabinoid percentage and also give you the percentages broken down into THC, CBD and CBN.

Gas Chromatography/Mass Spectrometry (GC-MS)

This method combines the features of gas chromatography alongside mass spectrometry to identify different substances within a test sample. GC with flame ionization or MS detection is now an established method for the analysis of cannabis. Derivatization (conversion into a derivative originating from the original to aid in identification) is necessary when information about cannabinoid acids and the dominating cannabinoids in the sample is required.

The total cannabinoid content, i.e. the amount of neutral cannabinoids plus the neutral cannabinoids formed by decarboxylation of the acidic cannabinoids, is determined when the GC analysis is performed without derivatization.

High Performance Liquid Chromatography (HPLC)

This is the most expensive but thorough test you can have performed on your samples. High-performance liquid chromatography allows the simultaneous determination of neutral and acidic phytocannabinoids without derivatization. Reversed phase columns and preferably solvent programmed gradient systems are used for the separation of major and minor cannabinoids and their corresponding acids for chemotyping (ratio acidic/neutral cannabinoids), studying the effect of manufacturing processes and storage conditions and batch comparison if required. Detection is usually performed by UV and diode array photometers, as well as by fluorescence, electrochemically and also MS.

The laboratory will send you a lab report detailing the overall cannabinoid content and the percentages of THC, CBD, et cetera. Depending on the type

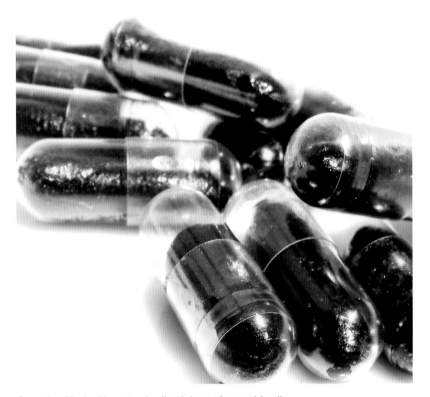

Capsules filled with a standardized dose of cannabis oil.

of testing you have had carried out the report may also include the terpene percentages and other information. The two main cannabinoids we are interested in are THC and CBD and in order to standardize the medications you are preparing obviously the overall percentage is required. For example, test results on the oil we produced from the Skunk Haze variety supplied to us by the CBD crew came back with an almost perfect 1:1 THC to CBD ratio and the overall active cannabinoid content was 80%. This allows us to accurately calculate the amount of cannabinoids we add to our preparations.

Calculating Dosage

After studying the laboratory report we were able to ascertain that our oil was the perfect cannabinoid profile that we required in order to make a generic copy of Sativex.

Signal 1: DAD1 A, Sig = 219,4 Ref = 450,80

RetTime (min)	Type	Area (mAU's)	Amt/Area	Amount (mg/g)	Grp	Name
2.707	VB	2.53031e4	3.15290e-5	398.89136		cbd
3.018		–	–	–		cbd-a
3.212	BB	92.00233	3.15290e-5	1.45037		cbg?
3.938	BV	3137.50562	1.79087e-5	20.09426		cbn
4.108	VB	487.65082	1.79089e-5	4.36665		cbn-a
4.636	VB	2.07813e4	3.18261e-5	330.69415		thc
5.481	VV	1039.76819	3.18259e-5	29.27612		thcv?
7.845	BV	352.15976	3.18254e-5	5.60381		thc-a

TOTALS: 1:1 oil   798.37673

Source: www.budbuddies.co.uk

The analysis report (below) shows that each gram of this oil contains 398.9 milligrams of CBD and 330.7 milligrams of THC.

Each bottle of Sativex contains 270 milligrams of CBD and 250 milligrams of THC, 680 milligrams of the Bud Buddies oil contains 271 milligrams of CBD and 225 milligrams of THC.

To administer 50 milligrams of CBD from the above oil you simply place

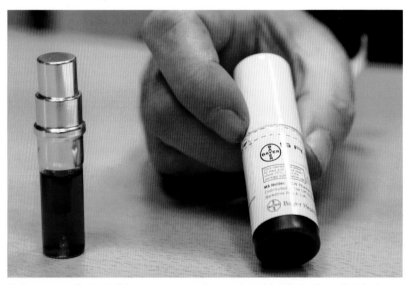

Sativex spray. To the left is a generic version produced by the authors that is far superior to Sativex and cost around $8.00 to produce.

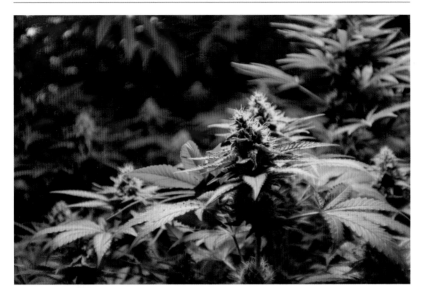

This grow room is producing some wonderful medication.

125 milligrams in a capsule. However, to administer smaller amounts it is beneficial to dilute the concentrated oil in non-psychoactive hemp or olive oil to act as a carrier.

One gram of the above oil contains 398 milligrams of CBD; therefore, if added to 10 grams of hemp seed oil or olive oil, each gram (1000 milligrams) would then contain 39.8 milligrams. If you place 0.5 gram (500 milligrams) of this oil into a capsule each one would contain 19.9 milligrams of CBD.

References

Introduction

1. "What is the lethal dose of marijuana? http://druglibrary.org/schaffer/library/mj_over-dose.htm

2. Quizlet, "BBH143: How Drugs Work", http://quizlet.com/19333522/bbh-143-how-drugs-work-flash-cards/

3. Peter Kershaw, *Economic Solutions: The Incredible Story of How You and America are Being Bankrupted & What You Can Do to Avoid the Wipeout,* (self-published, 1997), 29

4. "History of Marijuana as Medicine–2900 BC to Present", http://medicalmarijuana.procon.org/view.resource.php?resourceID=000143

5. "Reefer Madness", *The Economist,* April 27, 2006, http://www.economist.com/node/6849915

6. "Evidence Found of Ancient Marijuana Use", *Albany Times Union,* May 20, 1993, http://www.highbeam.com/doc/1G1-156697162.html

7. Leslie L. Iversen, *The Science of Marijuana Second Edition,* (USA: Oxford University Press, 2007), 116.

8. Gerald E. Wickens, *Economic Botany: Principles and Practices,* (Springer, 2004)

9. The Federal Observer, "Get Hemp to Jive, Man: Part II", http://www.federalobserver.com/archive.php?aid=2825

10. "Anslinger's Lies", http://www.ukcia.org/potculture/20/lies.html

11. "Prohibition Then and Now", notnowsilly.blogspot.com/2012/10/prohibition-then-and-now.html

12. "Mary Jane: Legal or Not?" http://33345569.nhd.weebly.com/why-marijuana-is-illegal.html

13. "Harry Anslinger Quotes", http://quotes.libertytree.ca/quote_blog/Harry.Anslinger.Quote.37DC14

14. "Mary Jane: Legal or Not?" http://33345569.nhd.weebly.com/why-marijuana-is-illegal.html

15. "Mary Jane: Legal or Not?" http://33345569.nhd.weebly.com/why-marijuana-is-illegal.html

16. "Why Hemp is Confused with Marijuana", http://marijuana-tax-act-1937.blogspot.com/

17. "Reefer Madness Propaganda Through the Ages", www.electricemporer.com/eecdrom/HTML/EMP/AA/ECH23.HTM

18. Wikipedia, en.wikipedia.org/wiki/Marihuana_Tax_Act_of_1937

19. I. Grant, et al, "Medical Marijuana: Clearing Away the Smoke", *The Open Neurology Journal* (2012), doi: 10.2174/1874205X01206010018

20. 'The Real Dope on Marinol and Sativex", www.tokeofthetown.com/2012/03/the_real_dope_on_marinol_and_sativex_bonus_stock_t.php

21. "Fibromyalgia and Medical Marijuana", www.webmd.com/fibromyalgia/guide/fibromyalgia-and-medical-marijuana

22. Wikipedia, en.wikipedia.org/wiki/United_States_v._Oakland_Cannabis_Buyers'_Cooperative

23. Wikipedia, http://en.wikipedia.org/wiki/Gonzales_v._Raich

24. FDA, "Inter-Agency Advisory Regarding Claims That Smoked Marijuana Is A Medicine", www.fda.gov/NewsEvents/Newsoom/PressAnnouncements/2006/ucm108643.htm

25. GW Pharmaceuticals, "Second Phase III Sativex Cancer Pain Trial Commences", www.gw-pharm.com/Second%20phase%20III%20Sativex%20cancer%20pain%20trial%20commences.aspx

26. Wikipedia, http://en.wikipedia.org/wiki/Nabilone

27. http://www.cesamet.com/patient-home.asp

28. "GW Pharmaceuticals GWP Exclusive License Agreement Signed With Novartis", www.bloomberg.com/apps/news?pid=newsarchive&sid=afJRuR74mwwY

29. "Novartis AG Pays GW Pharmaceuticals $5 Million Upfront for Sativex Rights in Multiple Territories", www.biospace.com/news_story.aspx?StoryID=216737&full=1

30. Steven Kotler, "Who Is Secretly Working to Keep

pot Illegal?" http://www.trutv.com/conspiracy/
in-the-shadows/pot-illegal/big-pharma-govern-
ment.html

31. Alex Berensen, "Hope, at $4,200 a Dose",
http://www.nytimes.com/2006/10/01/business/y
ourmoney/01drug.html?pagewanted=all&_r=0

32. United States Securities and Exchange Com-
mision, http://apps.shareholder.com/sec/view-
erContent.aspx?companyid=HNAB&docid=42
79385

33. http://www.google.com/patents/US6630507

34. "Pot Shrinks Tumors: Government Knew in '74",
http://americanmarijuana.org/pot.shrinks.tu-
mors.html

35. "Active Ingredient in Marijuana Kills Brain Cancer Kells, ABC News,
http://abcnews.go.com/Health/Healthday/story
?id=7235037&page=1

36. "Spain Study Confirms Hemp Oil Cures Cancer
Without Side Effects: http://www.endalldis-
ease.com/spain-study-confirms-hemp-oil-
cures-cancer-without-side-effects/

37: "Marijuana and Cancer: Scientists Find
Cannabis Compound Stops Metastasis in Aggressive Cancers", http://www.huffington-
post.com/2012/09/19/marijuana-and-cancer_n
_1898208.html

Chapter One: The Cannabis Plant

1. Wikipedia: http://en.wikipedia.org/wiki/Cannabis

2. Wikipedia: http://en.wikipedia.org/wiki/
Cannabaceae

3. "Improving the Quality of the Cannabis Debate:
Defining the Different Domains", http://www.
ncbi.nlm.nih.gov/pmc/articles/PMC1117366/

4. "Cannabinoids: The Active Ingredient of Marijuana", http://www.lycaeum.org/~sky/data/
grow/c2.html

5. "U of S Researchers Discover Cannabis
"Pharma Factory", University of Saskatchewan
On Campus News, http://news.usask.ca/
2012/07/16/u-of-s-researchers-discover-
cannabis-pharma-factory/

6. "The Health Benefits of Hemp Seeds (Plus a Raw
Eating Recipe)", http://cleancuisineand
more.com/health-benefits-of-hemp-seeds/

7. Wikipedia, http://en.wikipedia.org/wiki/Omega-
6_fatty_acid

8. "Omega 3 Fatty Acids", University of Maryland
Medical Center, http://www.umm.edu/altmed/
articles/omega-3-000316.htm

Chapter Two: How Cannabis Works

1. "How Drugs Affect Neurotransmitters", http://the-
brain.mcgill.ca/flash/i/i_03/i_03_m/i_03_m_par/i
_03_m_par_cannabis.html

2. "Anandamide",
http://www.princeton.edu/~achaney/tmve/wiki1
00k/docs/Anandamide.html

3. "Marinol vs. Natural Plant", NORML
http://norml.org/component/zoo/category/mari-
nol-vs-natural-cannabis

4. "Marijuana That Doesn't Get You Stoned",
http://news.discovery.com/tech/biotechnol-
ogy/medical-marijuana-thc-120706.htm

5. "Partnership For a Drug Free Amerca", http://
www.enotes.com/partnership-drug-free-amer-
ica-reference/partnership-drug-free-america

6. "David Nutt: My Views on Drug Classification",
The Guardian, http://www.guardian.co.uk/uk/
2009/nov/03/david-nutt-drugs-policy

7. F. M Lewke, et al, "Cannabidiol Enhances Anandamide Signaling and Alleviates Psychotic
Symptoms of Schizophrenia", Transl Psychiatry, v.2 (3) (2012), doi: 10.1038/tp.2012.15,
http://www.ncbi.nlm.nih.gov/pmc/articles/PM
C3316151/

8. "Marijuana: A Medical Marvel", http://www.the-
forbiddenknowledge.com/hardtruth/hemp_con-
spiracy.htm

9. Lynn E. Fiellin, et al, "Previous Use of Alcohol, Cigarettes, and Marijuana and Subsequent Abuse of
Prescription Opioids in Young Adults", Journal of
Adolescent Health, vol. 2 issue 2, 158-163, (February 2013) doi:10.1016/j.jadohealth.2012.06.010

10. Philip J. Hilts, "Relative Addictiveness of

Drugs", *New York Times*, (Aug 2, 1994) http://www.tfy.drugsense.org/tfy/addictvn.htm

11. "Gateway Theory", http://www.drugwarfacts.org/cms/?q=node/43#sthash.NkC4RGg7.dpbs

12. DA Simonetto, et al., "Cannabinoid Hyperemesis: A Case Series of 98 Patients", *Mayo Clinic Proceedings*, 87(2), 114-9 (February 2012), doi: 10.1016/j.mayocp.2011.10.005, http://www.ncbi.nlm.nih.gov/pubmed/22305024

13. "Torch the Joint", http://www.abc.net.au/unleashed/31556.html

14. "Marijuana Fact Sheet", www.whitehouse.gov/sites/.../marijuana_fact_sheet_jw_10-5-10.pdf

Chapter Three: Administration

1. "History of the Medical Use of Marijuana", http://www.skunked.co.uk/articles/marijuana-history.htm

2. W. B. O'Shaughnessy**, On the Preparations of the Indian Hemp, or Gunjah**, *Provincial Medical Journal and Retrospect of the Medical Sciences*, Vol. 5, No. 122 (Jan. 28, 1843), 343-347

3. "Subject: Medical Cannabis Use", http://www.new-territory.net/cann_uses.txt

4. "Pfizer, Set to Lose Lipitor, Feels No Pain With King Buy", Forbes (2012), http://www.forbes.com/2010/10/12/pfizer-king-acquisition-markets-equities-healthcare.html

5. "Eli Lilly and Cannabis", http://theweedscene.com/eli-lilly-and-cannabis/

6. Thomas w. Loker, *The History and Evolution of Healthcare in America: The Untold Backstory of Where We've Been, Where We Are, and Why Healthcare Needs Reform*, (iUniverse.com, 2012), 90

7. "A History of Cannabis Use for Stress and Depression: Rough Copies" http://www.cannabis-culture.com/node/24099

8. "Patented Pot vs. the Herbal Gold Standard", http://www.cannabisculture.com/node/19879

9. "Medical Cannabis DEA", http://www.scribd.com/doc/24836142/Medical-Cannabis-DEA-Judge-Francis-Young

10. "Florida Medical Examiners Commission 2008 Interim Report of Drugs Identified in Deceased Persons", http://web.docuticker.com/go/docubase/27642

11. "Prescription Drugs Kill 300 Percent More Americans Than Illegal Drugs", http://www.thebetter-healthstore.com/newsletter/11-13-08_November_05.html

12. "40,000 Deaths in USA Caused by Aspirin and Painkillers Every Year", http://adjusthealth.info/health-news/89-40000-deaths-in-usa-caused-by-aspirin-and-painkillers-every-year

13. "Short Lesson in Medicine", http://drsircus.com/medicine/short-lesson-in-medicine

14. Roman Bystrianyk, "Toxic and Deadly NSAIDS – An Investigative Report", http://www.healthsentinel.com/joomla/index.php?option=com_content&view=article&id=2446:toxic-and-deadly-nsaids&catid=39:reports&Itemid=52

15. Dr. Hilary Roberts, "Vitamin C: Linus Pauling Was Right All Along. A Doctor's Opinion", http://www.medicalnewstoday.com/releases/12154.php

16. American Cancer Society, http://www.cancer.org/treatment/treatmentsandsideeffects/complementaryandalternativemedicine/herbsvitamin-sandminerals/vitamin-c

17. "Chemo Can Damage Healthy Cells: Study", New Zealand Herald, http://www.nzherald.co.nz/lifestyle/news/article.cfm?c_id=6&objectid=10824989

18. "Chemotherapy Can Inadvertently Encourage Cancer Growth", http://www.medicalnewstoday.com/articles/248661.php

19. "Smoking Marijuana Not Bad for the Lungs", http://www.medicalnewstoday.com/articles/240146.php

20. "Study: Smoking Marijuana Not Linked With Lung Damage", http://healthland.time.com/2012/01/10/study-smoking-marijuana-not-linked-with-lung-damage/

21. "Study Finds No Cancer-Marijuana Connection", http://www.washingtonpost.com/wp-dyn/content/article/2006/05/25/AR2006052501729.html

22. "Pot's Active Ingredient Halts Lung Cancer Growth, Study Says", http://cannabisnews.com/news/22/thread22888.shtml

23 MA Elsohly, et al. "Rectal Bioavailability Of Delta-9-Tetrahydrocannabinol from the Hemisuccinate Ester in Monkeys", *Journal of Pharmaceutical Sciences*, 80(10) (Oct 1991), 942-5

24. "Collapse After Intravenous Injection of Hashish". http://www.ncbi.nlm.nih.gov/pmc/articles/PMC1986226/

25. Intravenous Marijuana Syndrome: Daniel Brandenburg, MD, Richard Wernick, MD.

Chapter Four: Cannabis Cures

1. "Corrie Yelland's Story", http://www.whale.to/cancer/corrie_yelland.html

2. Dr. Tod Mikuriya, "Cannabis as a Substitute for Alcohol a Harm Reduction Approach", http://harmreductioncenter.blogspot.com/2011/02/cannabis-as-substitute-for-alcohol-harm.html

3. "The History of Marijuana", http://www.michaelshouse.com/marijuana-rehab/history-of-marijuana/

4. "Alcohol and Public Health: Alcohol-Related Disease Impact", http://www.cdc.gov/alcohol/factsheets/alcohol-use.htm

5. "Alzheimer's to Triple by 2050 as Baby Boomers Age", http://www.reuters.com/article/2013/02/06/us-usa-alzheimers-idUSBRE9151AT20130206

6. "Marijuana's Active Ingredient Shown to Inhibit Primary Marker of Alzheimer's Disease", http://www.scripps.edu/news/press/2006/080906.html

7. D. Amtmann, et al., "Survey of Cannabis Use in Patients with Amyotrophic Lateral Sclerosis", *The American Journal of Hospice and Palliative Care*, 21(2) (Mar 2004), 95-104,

8. "Medicial Cannabis Helps ALS Patient Outlive Her Own Doctors", http://www.freedomisgreen.com/medical-cannabis-helps-als-patient-outlive-her-own-doctors/

9. "What is Zyprexa?". http://www.goodtherapy.org/drugs/zyprexa-olanzapine.html

10. "Cannabis May Help Anorexia", News.com.au, http://www.news.com.au/breaking-news/cannabis-may-help-anorexia/story-e6frfkp9-1111114332888

11. J Corey-Bloom, et al., "Smoked Cannabis for Spasticity in Multiple Sclerosis: A Randomized, Placebo-Controlled Trial", *Canadian Medical Association Journal*, 184(10), (July 2012), 1143-50, doi: 10.1503/cmaj.110837

12. "Mouse Model Links Alcohol Intake to Marijuana-Like Brain Compounds: New Pathway Presents Target for Medication Development", http://www.nih.gov/news/pr/jan2003/niaaa-20.htm

13. Yann le Strat and Bernard Le Foll, "Obesity and Cannabis Use: Results From 2 Representative National Surveys", *American Journal of Epidemiology*, (Aug 2011), doi: 10.1093/aje/kwr200

14. Richard A. Lovett, "Marijuana Has Anti-Inflammatory That Won't Get You High", National Geographic News, http://news.nationalgeo- graphic.com/news/2008/06/080624-marijuana.html

15. "Can Marijuana Help People with Asthma or Other Breathing Disorders?", http://medical-marijuana.procon.org/view.answers.php?questionID=000132

16. www.jddt.in/index.php/jddt/article/download/54/63

17. "More Diagnoses of Hyperactivity Causing Concern", New York Times, http://www.nytimes.com/2013/04/01/health/more-diagnoses-of-hyperactivity-causing-concern.html

18. Wikipedia: http://en.wikipedia.org/wiki/Methamphetamine

19. "ADHD Seems To Be Linked To Low Dopamine Brain Activity", http://www.medicalnewstoday.com/articles/79070.php

20. Steffens S, Mach F., "Cannabinoid Receptors in Atherosclerosis", Curr Opin Lipidol. 2006;17:519-526

21. "Effects of Cannabis Therapy on Endogenous Cannabinoids", http://www.cmcr.ucsd.edu/index.php?option=com_content&view=article&id=155:effects-of-cannabis-therapy-on-endogenous-cannabinoids&catid=41:research-studies&Itemid=135

22. "Why I Give My Autistic Son Pot, Part 4", http://www.slate.com/articles/double_x/double x/2011/05/why_i_give_my_autistic_son_pot_pa rt_4.html

23. "Cannabis Enhances Bipolar Patients' Neurocognitive Performance", http://www.med-icalnewstoday.com/articles/249006.php

24. "Active Ingredient in Marijuana Kills Brain Cancer Cells", http://abcnews.go.com/Health/ Healthday/story?id=7235037&page=1

25. "Chemotherapy Can Do More Harm Than Good", http://articles.mercola.com/sites/arti-cles/archive/2008/12/02/chemotherapy-can-do-more-harm-than-good.aspx

26. "Cancer Chemotherapy Backfires", http:// www.natureasia.com/en/research/highlight/1822

27. Dr. Christina Davis, et al. "Long-term effects of continuing adjuvant tamoxifen to 10 years versus stopping at 5 years after diagnosis of oestrogen receptor-positive breast cancer: ATLAS, a randomised trial", The Lancet, Vol. 381, issue 9869, (Mar 2013), doi:10.1016/S0140-6736(12)61963-1

28. Redmond CK, Wickerham DL, Cronin W, et al., "The NSABP breast cancer prevention trial (BCPT): a progress report." [Abstract] Proceedings of the American Society of Clinical Oncology 12: A-78, 69, 1993.

29. "IVAX Ges US Go-Ahead for Generic Novaldex", http://www.thepharmaletter.com/file/83790/ivax -gets-us-go-ahead-for-generic-nolvadex.html

30. Betty Martini, "Tamoxifen, Tears and Terror", http://www.holisticmed.com/toxic/tamoxifen.shtml

31. "Health Fears Over Cancer Drug", BBC News, http://news.bbc.co.uk/2/hi/health/466134.stm

32. Dr. Christina Davis, et al. "Long-term effects of continuing adjuvant tamoxifen to 10 years versus stopping at 5 years after diagnosis of oestrogen receptor-positive breast cancer: ATLAS, a randomised trial", The Lancet, Vol. 381, issue 9869, (Mar 2013), doi:10.1016/S0140-6736(12)61963-1

33. www.sciencenews.org/pages/pdfs/data/ 1996/149-09/14909-03.pdf

34. Betty Martini, "Tamoxifen, Tears and Terror", http://www.holisticmed.com/toxic/tamoxifen.shtml

35. "Cannabis Compound Stops Spread of Breast Cancer: Researchers", CBC News, http://www.cbc.ca/news/health/story/2007/11/ 19/cannabis-cancer.html

36. www.nel.edu/pdf_/25_12/NEL251204R02_ Russo_.pdf

37. L. Degenhardt, et al., "The relationship between cannabis use, depression and anxiety among Australian adults: findings from the National Survey of Mental Health and Well-Being.", Social Psychiatry and Psychiatric Epidemiology, 36(5) (May 2001), 219-227

38. Tina Minkowitz, "The U.N. Asks the U.S. to Defend its Use of Forced Psychiatric Drugging", http://www.madinamerica.com/2013/04/un-asks-the-united-states-to-defend-its-practice-of-forced-psychiatric-drugging/

39. "Study in Mice Shows Why Antidepressants Often Fail", http://www.foxnews.com/story/ 2010/01/14/study-in-mice-shows-why-antide-pressants-often-fail/

40. "Cannabis: Potent Anti-Depressant In Low Doses, Worsens Depression At High Doses", http://www.sciencedaily.com/releases/2007/10/ 071023183937.htm

41. A. Chaterjee, et al., "A dramatic response to inhaled cannabis in a woman with central thalamic pain and dystonia", Journal of Pain and Symptom Management, 24(1) (July 2002), 4-6,

42. www.ncbi.nlm.nih.gov/pubmed/17952650

43. "Hepatitis C Now Kills More Americans Than HIV", http://health.usnews.com/health-news/news/articles/2012/02/20/hepatitis-c-now-kills-more-americans-than-hiv

44. http://www.hepatitis-central.com/mt/archives/ 2007/06/the_pros_and_co.html

45. "AIDS Patient Turns to Medical Marijuana for Relief", http://www.herbal-smoke.net/aids-pa-tient-turns-to-medical-marijuana-for-relief/

46. P. Conroe, et al., "Controlled clinical trial of

References

cannabidiol in Huntington's disease", *Pharmacology, Biochemistry and Behavior*, 40(3) (Nov 1991), 701-708

47. www.qahda.com/HQ_Newsletter_July_2011.pdf

48. "Alternative therapies for overactive bladder: Cannabis and urge incontinence", link.springer.com/article/10.1007%2Fs11884-008-0033-4

49. "Mouse Model Links Alcohol Intake to Marijuana-Like Brain Compounds New Pathway Presents Target for Medication Development", http://www.nih.gov/news/pr/jan2003/niaaa-20.htm

50. Yann le Strat and Bernard Le Foll, "Obesity and Cannabis Use: Results From 2 Representative National Surveys", *American Journal of Epidemiology*, (Aug 2011), doi: 10.1093/aje/kwr200

51. Robert J. McKallip, et al., "Cannabidiol-Induced Apoptosis in Human Leukemia Cells: A Novel Role of Cannabidiol in the Regulation of p22^{phox}and Nox4 Expression", *Molecular Pharmacology* vol. 70 no.3 (Sep 2006), 897-908,

52. "Chemicals in Cannabis May Fight MRSA", http://www.webmd.com/news/20080904/marijuana-chemicals-may-fight-mrsa

53. "Multiple Sclerosis and Extract of Cannabis (MUSEC): a randomised, double-blind, placebo-controlled phase III trial to determine the efficacy and safety of a standardised oral extract of Cannabis sativa for the symptomatic relief of muscle stiffness and pain in Multiple Sclerosis (MS)", http://www.controlled-trials.com/ISRCTN42223114

54. J Corey-Bloom, et al., "Smoked Cannabis for Spasticity in Multiple Sclerosis: A Randomized, Placebo-Controlled Trial", *Canadian Medical Association Journal*, 184(10), (July 2012), 1143-50, doi: 10.1503/cmaj.110837

55. "Study: Cannabis Extracts Mitigate Muscle Stiffness in Multiple Sclerosis Patients", http://norml.org/news/2012/07/26/study-cannabis-extracts-mitigate-muscle-stiffness-in-multiple-sclerosis-patients

56. cannabis.cluster005.ovh.net/data/pdf/2001-01-1.pdf

57. "Medical Marijuana Possible Treatment for Osteoporosis", http://naturalsociety.com/medical-marijuana-possible-treatment-osteoporosis/

58. http://norml.org/library/item/osteoporosis

59. "More Than Five Million Americans Abuse Painkillers Every Month". http://www.besmartbewell.com/media/painkillers.htm

60. "Medicinal Marijuana Effective for Neuropathic Pain in HIV", http://ucsdnews.ucsd.edu/newsrel/health/08-08MedMarijHIV.asp

61. cannabis.cluster005.ovh.net/data/pdf/2001-01-1.pdf

62. med.org/studies/ww_en_db_study_show.php?s_id=14

63. www.cannabisculture.com/content/.../WhiteHouse-No-Marijuana-PTSD

64. www.ptsd.va.gov/professional/newsletters/research.../V20N1.pdf

65. "Generic OxyContin Pains the FDA", http://online.wsj.com/article/SB10001424127887327434580457842269180585 1784.html

66. "Suicide Among War Veterans is a Scourge of Military Conflicts", http://www.open.ac.uk/platform/blogs/society-matters/suicide-among-war-veterans-scourge-military-conflicts

67. "U.S. Army Suicides Rising Sharply, Study Finds", http://health.usnews.com/health-news/news/articles/2012/03/08/us-army-suicides-rising-sharply-study-finds

68. http://homecomingvets.com/

69. Melanie C. Dreher, et al., "Prenatal Marijuana Exposure and Neonatal Outcomes in Jamaica: An Ethnographic Study", *Pediatrics*, 93(2) (Feb 1994), 254-260

70. "Cannabinoids, Like Those Found in Marijuana, Occur Naturally in Human Breast Milk", http://www.naturalnews.com/036526_cannabinoids_breast_milk_THC.html

71. "CN BC: Marijuana Effective Against Morning Sickness: Study", http://www.mapinc.org/drugnews/v05/n1583/a06.html?269296

72. Ferrari F, Ottani A, Giuliani D., "Inhibitory effects of the cannabinoid agonist HU 210 on rat sexual behaviour", *Physiology and Behavior* 69 (2000); 547–554

73. "Cannabis Plays Havoc With Men's Orgasms", http://www.latrobe.edu.au/news/articles/2009/article/cannabis-plays-havoc-with-mens-orgasms

74. "Cannabis-like Cream Effective Combating Pruritus, Stidy Says", http://norml.org/news/2005/12/15/cannabis-like-cream-effective-combating-pruritus-study-says

75. E. Del-Bel, et al., "Cannabidiol-treated rats exhibited higher motor score after cryogenic spinal cord injury", *Neurotoxicity Research* 21(3), (Apr 2012), 271-280, doi: 10.1007/s12640-011-9273-8.

76. "Report Highlights Danger of Irish-Grown Cannabis", http://www.coloradodispensaryproducts.com/tag/cbd/

77. "Cannabinoid Improves Locomotor Function, Reducse Injury in Animal Model of Spinal Cord Injury", http://norml.org/news/2011/11/17/cannabinoid-improves-locomotor-function-reduces-injury-in-animal-model-of-spinal-cord-injury

78. "Federal Study Suggests Marijuana May Prevent Brain Damage in Stroke Victims", http://stopthedrugwar.org/chronicle-old/049/study.shtml

79. K.R. Muller-Vahl, "Cannabinoids Reduce Symptoms of Tourette's Syndrome", *Expert Opinion on Pharmacotherapy*, 4(10) (Oct 2003), 1717-1725,

80. Clare M. Eddy and Hugh E. Rickards, "Treatment Strategies for Tics in Tourette Syndrome", *Therapeutic Advances in Neurological Disorders* 4(1) (Jan 2011), 25-45, doi: 10.1177/1756285610390261

Chapter Six: Hemp Nutrition and Health

1. http://www.fuelrunning.com/quotes/2013/01/10/the-problem-is-we-are-not-eating-food-anymore-we-are-eating-food-like-products-dr-alejandro-junger-hungry-for-change-film/

2. www.who.int/entity/dietphysicalactivity/media/en/gsfs_obesity.pdf

3. "Does Adaptation to a Global Life Explain the "Obesity Epidemic"?, http://blogs.lse.ac.uk/healthandsocialcare/2013/04/16/does-adaptation-to-a-global-life-explain-the-obesity-epidemic/

4. "Landmark Reprot: Excess Body Fat Causes Cancer", http://preventcancer.aicr.org/site/News2?page=NewsArticle&id=12898&news_iv_ctrl=0&abbr=pr_

5. Chris Conrad, *Hemp for Health; The Medical and Nutritional Uses of Cannabis Sativa*, (UK; Healing Arts Press 1997)

6. "Shelled Hemp Seed". http://www.uofmhealth.org/health-library/hn-4393002

7. J. Luo et al.,"Extract from Fructus cannabis activating calcineurin improved learning and memory in mice with chemical drug-induced dysmnesia"; *Acta Pharmacologica Sinica* 24(11) (2003), 1137-1142

8. "Shelled Hemp Seed", http://www.uofmhealth.org/health-library/hn-4393002#hn-4393002-uses

9. "Is Juicing Raw Cannabis the Miracle Health Cure That Some of its Proponents Believe it to Be?" http://www.alternet.org/personal-health/juicing-raw-cannabis-miracle-health-cure-some-its-proponents-believe-it-be

10. "Why The Raw Cannabis Juicing Trend May Not Be all its Juiced Up To Be", http://boingboing.net/2012/01/10/why-the-raw-cannabis-juicing.html

11. "Cannabis Compound May Stop Metastatic Breast Cancer", http://abcnews.go.com/Health/Healthday/story?id=4509456&page=2

12. S.Takeda, et al., "Cannabidiolic acid, a major cannabinoid in fiber-type cannabis, is an inhibitor of MDA-MB-231 breast cancer cell migration", *Toxicology Letters*, 214(3), (Nov 2012), 314-319, doi: 10.1016/j.toxlet.2012.08.029

Appendix 1: Cancer-Fighting Foods

1. "Dairy Products Increase Risk of Prostate Cancer", http://www.pcrm.org/health/mednews/dairy-products-increase-risk-of-prostate-cancer

Bibliography

Agurell S., H. Halldin, JE. Lindgren, A. Ohlsson, M. Widman, H. Gillespie and LE. Hollister. 1986. Pharmacokinetics and metabolism of delta-1-tetrahydrocannabinol and other cannabinoids with emphasis on man. Pharmacological Rev 38:21-43.

AMA Council on Scientific Affairs. 1980. Marihuana reconsidered: Pulmonary risks and therapeutic potentials. Conn Med 44:521-523.

AMA Council on Scientific Affairs. 1981. Marijuana. Its health hazards and therapeutic potentials. J Amer Med Assoc 248:1823-1827.

Anja Huizink and Eduard Mulder. 2005. Maternal smoking, drinking or cannabis use during pregnancy and neurobehavioral and cognitive functioning in human offspring. Neuroscience and Biobehavioral Reviews 30: 1-18.

Awad AB, Fink CS. Phytosterols as anticancer dietary components: Evidence and mechanism of action. J Nutr 130:2127-30, 2000.

Balle et al. 1999. Cannabis and pregnancy. Ugeskr Laeger 161: 5024-5028.

Barofsky, P. Simon, and S. Rosenberg. 1979. Delta-9-tetrahydrocannabinol as antiemetic in cancer patients receiving high-dose methotrexate; a prospective, randomized evaluation. Ann Int Med 91:819-824.

Beal JE, R. Olson, L. Laubenstein, J.O. Morales, P. Bellamen, B. Yangco. 1995.

Bhargava HN. 1978. Potential therapeutic application of naturally occurring and synthetic cannabinoids. General Pharmacol 9:195-213.

Birch, E.A. 1889. The use of Indian hemp in the treatment of chronic chloral and chronic opium poisoning. Lancet Vol. 1:625.

Bosy TZ, Cole KA. Consumption and quantitation of D9 tetrahydrocannabinol in commercially available hemp seed oil products. Anal Toxicol, 7:562-6, 2000.

Brousseau ME, Schaefer EJ. Diet and Coronary Heart Disease: Clinical Trials. Curr Atheroscler Rep 2:487-493, 2000.

Cannabinoids and Glioma's. Velasco G, Carracedo A, Blázquez C, Lorente M, Aguado T, Haro A, Sánchez C, Galve-Roperh I, Guzmán M. PMID: 17952650 [PubMed – indexed for MEDLINE]

Clifford, D.B. 1983. Tetrahydrocannabinol for tremor in multiple sclerosis. Annals Neurol 13(6), 669-671.

Consroe, P., R. Musty, J. Rein, W. Tillery and R. Pertwee. 1997. The perceived effects of smoked cannabis on patients with multiple sclerosis. European Neurology 38(1):44-48.

Consroe, P., R. Sandyk and S.R. Snider. 1986. Open label evaluation of cannabidiol in dystonic movement disorder. Intern J Neuroscience 30:277-282.

Consroe, PF, G.C. Wood and H. Buchsbaum. 1975. Anticonvulsant effect of marihuana smoking. J Amer Med Assoc 234:306-307.

Cooler, P. and J.M. Gregg. 1977. Effect of delta-9-tetrahydrocannabinol on intraocular pressure in humans. South Med J 70:951-954.

Corey-Bloom J, et al. Smoked cannabis for spasticity in multiple sclerosis: a randomized, placebo-controlled trial

Cousens, K. and A. Dimascio. 1973. Delta-9-THC as an hypnotic. An experimental study of 3 dose levels. Psychopharmacologia 33:355-364.

Cunha, J.M., E.A. Carlini, A.E. Periera, O.L. Ramos, C. Pimental, R. Gagliardi, W.L. Snavito, N. Lander and R. Mechoulam. 1980. Chronic administration of cannabidiol to healthy volunteers and epileptic patients. Pharmacology 21:175-185.

DeLuca P, Rothman D, Zurier RB. Marine and botanical lipids as immunomodulatory and therapeutic agtents in the treatment of rheumatoid arthritis. Rheum Dis Clin N Am 21:759-77.

Doblin, R.E. and M.A.R. Kleiman. 1991. Marijuana as antiemetic medicine: A survey of oncologist's experiences and attitudes. J Clin Oncol 313-319.

Dreher et al. 1994. Prenatal marijuana exposure and neonatal outcomes in Jamaica: An ethnographic study. Pediatrics 93: 254-260.

Dronabinol as a treatment for anorexia associated with weight loss in patients with AIDS. J Pain Symptom Manage 10:89-97.

Dunn, M. and R. Davis. 1974. The perceived effects of marijuana on spinal cord injured males. Paraplegia 12(3):175-178.

Eaton SB, Eaton III SB, Konner MJ. Paleolithic nutrition revisited: A twelve-year retrospective on its nature and implications. Eur J Clin Nutr 51:207-216, 1997.

Ekert, H., K.D. Waters, I.A. Julik, J. Mobina and P. Lougnnan. 1979. Amelioration of cancer chemotherapy-induced nausea and vomiting by delta-9-tetrahydrocannabinol.

English et al. 1997. Maternal cannabis use and birth weight: a meta-analysis. Addiction 92: 1553-1560.

Ethan Russo. 2002. Cannabis Treatments in Obstetrics and Gynecology: A Historical Review. Journal of Cannabis Therapeutics 2: 5-35.

Fan YY, Ramos KS, Chapkin RS. Modulation of atherosclerosis by dietary gamma-linolenic acid. Adv Exp Med Biol 469:485-91, 1999.

Fenstrom JD. Effects of dietary polyunsaturated fatty acids on neuronal function. Lipids 34:161-9, 1999.

Fergusson et al. 2002. Maternal use of cannabis and pregnancy outcome. BLOG: An International Journal of Obstetrics and Gynaecology 109: 21-27.

Fishbein, M. 1942. Migraine associated with menstruation. Journal of the American Medical Association Vol. 120: 4, 326.

Goldschmidt et al. 2008. Prenatal marijuana exposure and intelligence test performance at age 6. Journal of the American Academy of Child Adolescent Psychiatry 47: 254-263.

Goodman, L.S. & Gilman, A. (Eds.). 1955. The Pharmacological Basis of Therapeutics. New York: Macmillan.

Hare, H.A. 1887. Clinical and physiological notes on the action of cannabis indica. Therapeutic Gazette Vol. 11; 225-228.

Hornstra G, Kester AD. Effect of the dietary fat type on arterial thrombosis tendency: systemic studies with a rat model. Atherosclerosis 131:25-33, 1997.

Horrobin DF. Essential fatty acid metabolism and its modification in atopic eczema. J Am Clin Nutr 71:367S-72S, 2000.

John P. Morgan and Lynn Zimmer. Intravenous Marijuana Syndrome: Daniel Brandenburg, MD, Richard Wernick, MD. Marijuana Myths, Marijuana Facts: A Review of the Scientific Evidence. New York: The Lindesmith Center. 1997.

Kang JX, Leaf A. Prevention of fatal cardiac arrhymias by polyunsaturated fatty acids. Amer J Clin Nutr, 71:202S-207S, 2000.

Kenny FS, Pinder SE, Ellis IO, et. al. Gamma-linolenic acid with tamoxifen as primary therapy in breast cancer. Int J Cancer 85:643-8, 2000.

Kris-Etherton PM, Taylor DS, Yu-Poth S et. al. Polyunsaturated fatty acids in the food chain in the United States. Am J Clin Nutr, 71:179S-88S 2000.

Kruger MC, Coetzer H, Winter R, et. al. Calcium, gamma-linolenic acid and eicosapentaneoic acid supplementation in senile osteoporosis. Aging 10:385-94, 1998.

Leson G, Pless P, Grotenherman F, Kalant H, El-Sohly MA. Food products from hemp seeds: Could their consumption interfere with workplace drug testing J Anal Toxicol, Accepted, 2000.

Leventhal LJ, Boyce EG, Zurier, RB. Treatment of arthritis with gamma-linolenic acid. Ann Intern Med 119:876-873, 1993.

Li H. "The Origin and Use of Cannabis in Eastern Asia: Their Linguistic Cultural Implications," in Cannabis and Culture, ed. V Rubin, The Hague: Mouton, 1975.

Loewe, S. 1950. The active principles of cannabis and the pharmacology of the cannabinols. Archiv fur Experimentale Pathologie und Pharmakologie Vol. 211: 175-193.

Marshall, C.R. 1898. A contribution to the pharmacology of cannabis indica. Journal of the American Medical Association Vol. 31: 882-891.

Mattison, J.B. 1891. Cannabis indica as an anodyne and hypnotic. St. Louis Medical and Surgical Journal Vol. 61: 265-271.

Mayor's Committee on Marihuana. 1944. The Marihuana Problem in the City of New York. Lancaster, Pennsylvania: Jacques Cattell Press.

McMeens, R.R. 1860. Report of the Ohio State Medical Committee on cannabis indica. Transactions of the Fifteenth Annual Meeting of the Ohio State Medical Society. Columbus: Follett, Foster & Co., pp. 75-100.

Moghadasian MH, Frohlich JJ. Effects of dietary phytosterols on cholesterol metabolism and atherosclerosis: Clinical and experimental evidence. Amer J Med 107:588-94, 1999.

Nadkarni, A. (Ed.). 1954. Indian Materia Medica. Bombay: Popular Book Depot.

O'Shaughnessy, W.B. 1838-40. On the preparations of the Indian hemp, or gunjah. Transactions of the Medical and Psychical Society of Bengal. pp. 71-102.

Peter Fried. 1995. Prenatal exposure to marihuana and tobacco during infancy, early and middle childhood: effects and an attempt at synthesis. Archives of Toxicology Supplement 17: 233-260.

Peter Fried. 2002. Conceptual issues in behavior teratology and their application in determining long-term sequelae of prenatal marihuana exposure. Journal of Child Psychology and Psychiatry 43: 81-102.

PubMed: "Acta Pharmacologica Sinica;" Extract from Fructus cannabis activating calcineurin improved learning and memory in mice with chemical drug-induced dysmnesia; J. Luo et al.; 2003.

Reynolds, J.R. 1890. Therapeutic uses and toxic effects of cannabis indica. Lancet Vol. 1: 637-638.

Richardson et al. 1995. Prenatal alcohol, marijuana and tobacco use: infant mental and motor development. Neurotoxicology and Teratology 17: 479-487.

Rizzo MT, Regazzi E, Garau D, et. al. Induction of apoptosis by arachodonic acid in chronic myeloid leukemia cells. Cancer Res 59:5047-53, 1999.

Robbins M, Ali K, McCaw R, et. al. Gamma-linolenic acid-mediated cytotoxicity in human prostate cancer cells. Adv Exp Med Biol 469:499-504, 1999.

Singh Gurkirpal, MD, "Recent Considerations in Nonsteroidal Anti-Inflammatory Drug Gastropathy", The American Journal of Medicine, July 27, 1998, p. 31S.

Siscovic DS, Raghunathan TE, King I et. al. Dietary intake of long-chain n-3 polyunsaturated fatty acids and the risk of primary cardiac arrest. Amer J Clin Nutr, 71:208S-212S, 2000.

Southgate J, Pitt E, Trejdosiewicz LK. The effects of dietary fatty acids on the proliferation of normal human urothelial cells in vitro. Br J Cancer 74:728-34, 1996.

Trivers et al. 2006. Parental marijuana use and risk of childhood acute myeloid leukaemia: a report from the Children's Cancer Group. Pediatric and Perinatal Epidemiology 20: 110-118.

University of Maryland Medical Center: Omega 3 Fatty Acids

University of Michigan: Shelled Hemp Seeds.

Vartek S, Robbins ME, Spector AA. Polyunsaturated fatty acids increase the sensitivity of 36B10 rat astrocytoma cells to radiation-induced cell kill. Br J Cancer 77:1612-20, 1998.

Walton, R.P. 1938. Marihuana: America's New Drug Problem. Philadelphia: J.B. Lippincott.

Waring, E.J. 1874. Practical Therapeutics: Articles of the Materia Medica. Philadelphia: Lindsay & Blakiston. pp. 157-161.

Wei-Ni Lin Curry. 2002. Hyperemesis Gravidarum and clinical cannabis: To eat or not to eat? Journal of Cannabis Therapeutics 2: 63-83.

Westfall et al. 2006. Survey of medicinal cannabis use among childbearing women: Patterns of its use in pregnancy and retroactive self-assessment of its efficacy against 'morning sickness.'

Complementary Therapies in Clinical Practice 12: 27-33.

Wolfe M. MD, Lichtenstein D. MD, and Singh Gurkirpal, MD, "Gastrointestinal Toxicity of Nonsteroidal Anti-inflammatory Drugs", The New England Journal of Medicine, June 17, 1999, Vol. 340, No. 24, pp. 1888-1889.

Wright S. Essential fatty acids and the skin. Br J Derm 125:503-515, 1991.

Yehuda S, Rabinovitz S, Carrasso RL, Mostofsky DI. Essential fatty acids preparation (SR-3) improves Alzheimer's patients quality of life. Int J Neurosci 87:141-9, 1996.

Youdim KA, Martin A, Joseph JA. Essential fatty acids and the brain: possible health implications. Int J Dev Neurosci 18:383-99, 2000.

Yu Y. Agricultural history over seven thousand years in China, In: Feeding a Billion: Frontiers of Chinese Agriculture, ed. S Witter, 1987.

Zammit et al. 2009. Maternal tobacco, cannabis and alcohol use during pregnancy and risk of adolescent psychotic symptoms in offspring. The British Journal of Psychiatry 195: 294-300.

Zurier RB, Rossetti RG, Jacobson EW, et. al. gamma-linolenic acid treatment of rheumatoid arthritis. A randomized, placebo-controlled trial. Arthritis Rheum 39:1808-17, 1996.

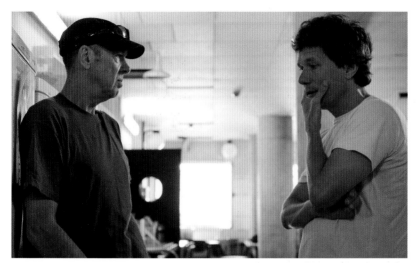

Professor Manuel Guzman (right): "You [Jeff] are combining what you see in the clinics with the best in the research field with the needs of cancer patients and you put that information together in a rational manner and I also think in a very valuable manner."

About the Authors

Jeff Ditchfield is a successful author, outspoken campaigner and activist. He was one of the original founders of Bud Buddies, an organization that supplied cannabis free of charge for medicinal users from 2002 to 2007. His organization was a nonprofit venture that was operated out of medical necessity, yet he was eventually prosecuted for supplying cannabis. After a lengthy trial he was found not guilty by a jury of his peers. However, this angered the authorities so much that they took the case to the Court of Appeal and he was unconstitutionally declared guilty despite the jury's lawful decision to acquit him. Undeterred, Jeff sent every member of the U.K. government a cannabis plant and drug tested a Chief Constable who reluctantly agreed whilst giving a press interview. Jeff has lectured at The Royal College of General Practitioners and John Moores University on the medicinal application of cannabis and is the former proprietor of The Beggars Belief, the first cannabis coffee shop in Wales. Jeff is internationally acclaimed and respected for his research and testing of cannabis-based oils and preparations for medical use.

Mel Thomas is a former commercial grower who was one of the first to introduce Skunk cannabis to the U.K. It was in Holland that he first learned how to make cannabis oil and perfected the art over many years. Eventually arrested he was charged with producing skunk cannabis valued at £2.8 million; the trial judge called him, "A horticultural expert involved in a resolute and successful attempt to produce cannabis on a commercial scale." Convicted of producing cannabis he was sentenced to five years imprisonment and held as a category "A" prisoner on a maximum-security wing in one of Europe's most secure jails. Mel also campaigns against cannabis prohibition and his first book, *Cannabis Cultivation* has now been in print for over ten years, being one of the top five best-selling cultivation books ever written. As well as radio show appearances Mel has written numerous articles for *Skunk* magazine, *Releaf, Weed World, Cannabis Culture* and *Grow Magazine* based in Germany and is an outspoken critic of the pharmaceutical industry and government policies, particularly as two family members suffer from conditions that cannabis can alleviate; namely multiple sclerosis and Parkinson's syndrome.

Index